Two Fat Mice
and the
Fork in the Road

Two Fat Mice and the Fork in the Road
Copyright © 2018 By Michael Dalk

ISBN-13: 978-0-9985261-0-2

www.WeightLossRd.com

Printed in the United States of America

A story about

Two Fat Mice and the Fork in the Road

by

Michael Dalk

The Fork in the Road.

Contents

Tools Needed

1. Leverage on yourself to change
2. A good attitude
3. A digital scale that measures body fat
4. A cloth tape measure
5. A calculator
6. A camera
7. Access to the internet
8. Comfortable shoes
9. Food scale
10. Measuring cups and spoons

The Fork in the Road.

One day, on Weight Loss Road, two mice begin a journey to lose weight. These mice have very different reasons for choosing to lose weight. Truly Try gained weight over the years but is sure she can lose the weight for an upcoming wedding. Dewey Do has been overweight most of his life and is skeptical about dieting because he has tried every diet out there and wonders why he gains the weight back after losing it.

Weight Loss Road is a long, windy road with many twists and turns. Down its well-traveled roads and newly paved paths, are two travelers who come across familiar and unique challenges. If you dare to join these mice, their journey might surprise you.

Dewey Do invited Truly on this journey. During a conversation, Dewey mentions to Truly about a friend, Olive the owl, who traveled this road and lost weight. Olive was initially apprehensive about showing Dewey the road, but she eventually did. She knew this journey would be difficult, so she told Dewey to bring a friend for support.

"I'm glad you invited me along," Truly said. "I've got to lose weight before I go to a wedding. What did your friend tell you about this road?"

"She told me it's important to be committed to the journey. So, before she would show me this road, I had to convince her I was committed. I'm happy you're able to come, I was nervous to start this journey alone."

"No reason to be nervous, we can lose weight. Your friend Olive lost weight and so can we. What we need is a new diet and we will both lose weight quickly."

"I don't know Truly, I've tried every diet out there. I lose weight, only to gain it back, I need to do something different. I hope this road will help me understand why I keep gaining the weight back after I lose it."

Truly jumps around with excitement as they travel along the smooth beginning of the Road.

"I can't wait to lose weight. Do you think this road will be easy? We're going to drop some serious pounds, I know it."

"Whoa, slow down Truly. I don't think this road will be easy. I've tried many of these new diets and there hard to maintain. I keep hearing good things about Weight Loss Road and Olive was very successful. I think we can do this."

"Come on Dewey, let's hurry and see where this road will lead us."

After walking a while, both mice come to the fork in the
road with two different ways to go. In front of each road
are signs describing the road ahead.

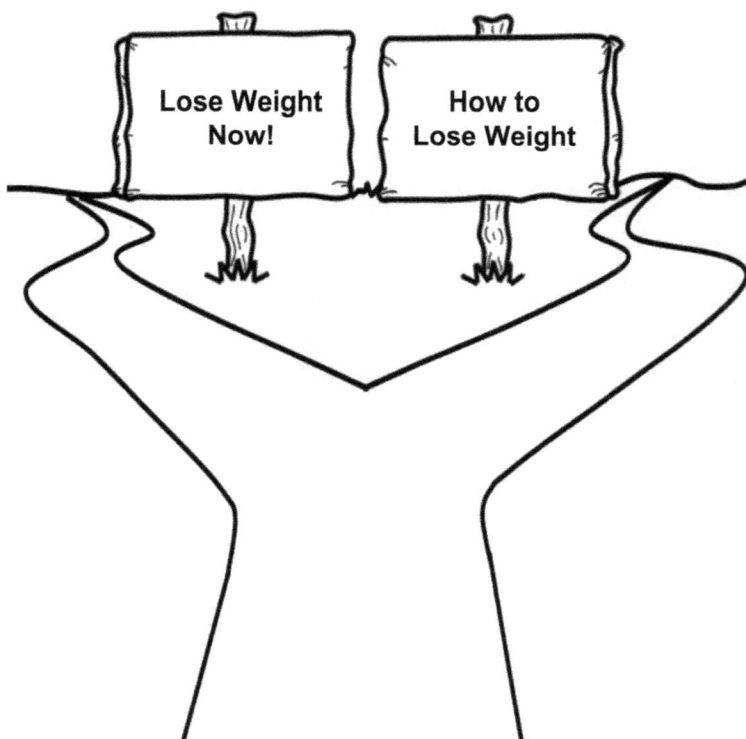

Lose Weight Now!

How to Lose Weight

Truly reads the sign on the left road and says, "Lose Weight Now! That's the way we should go."

"That way seems familiar," Dewey said, "I need to do something different. Let's think about this."

"What's there to think about?" We both want to 'lose weight now' and I have a wedding to go to."

"You can go ahead Truly, I'll catch up."

"Alright, I'll see you later."

Truly hurries down this well-traveled road, excited with the promise of losing weight.

Dewey reads both signs:

Lose Weight Now! How to Lose Weight.

He thinks for a moment:

If I learn how to lose weight maybe I'll also learn why I keep gaining it back. I usually just try a new diet, so educating myself first will be different. I think I will learn how to lose weight.

Dewey stumbles as he starts up the newly paved path.

Truly hurrying down the well-traveled road, excited to lose some weight, sees a sign with a new diet to help her lose weight.

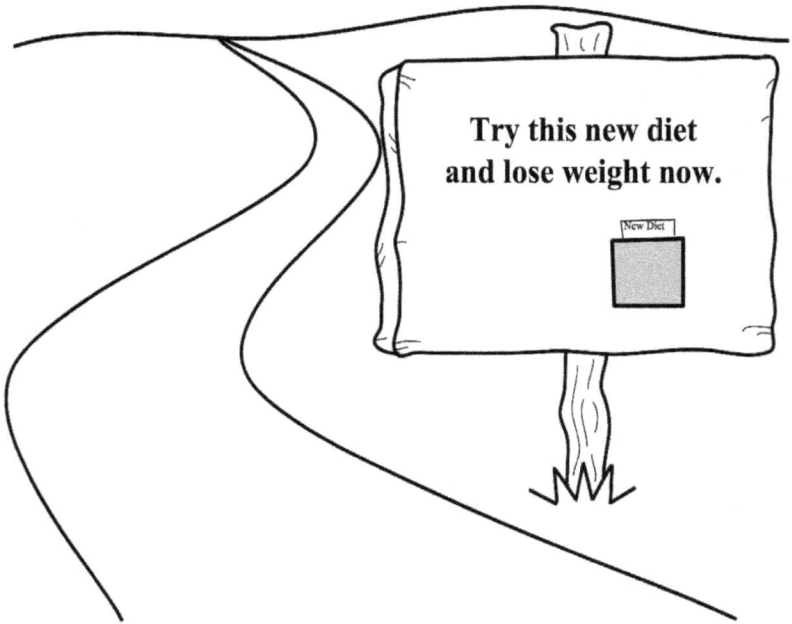

Truly reads the sign and as she grabs a pamphlet, thinks: *This new diet will be perfect. I'm going to try this new diet and lose weight now. I will be ready in no time for that wedding.*

Truly runs off and starts the new diet, as the road begins up a hill.

Dewey heads up a slight grade on what looks like a long path. He sees a sign that says to commit.

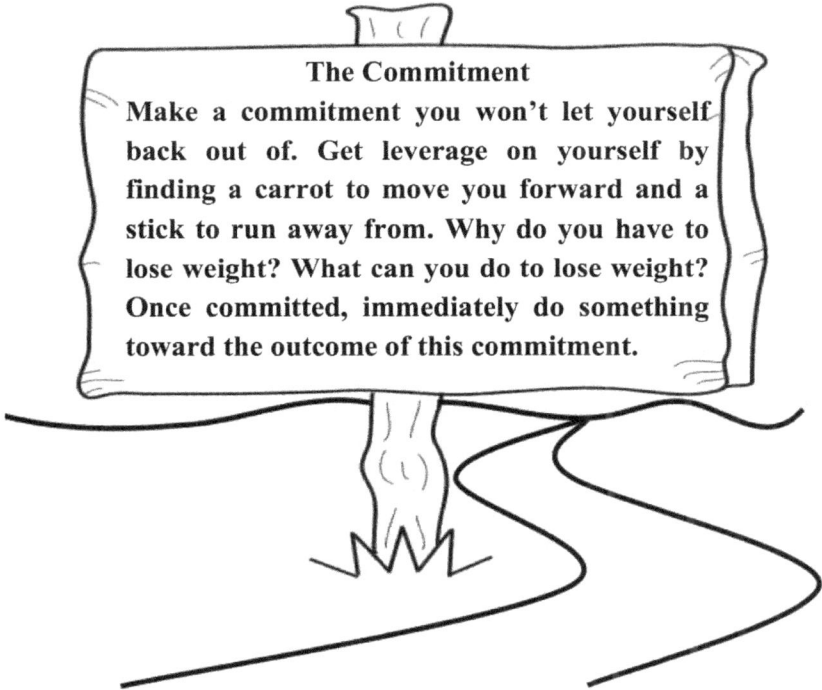

The Commitment
Make a commitment you won't let yourself back out of. Get leverage on yourself by finding a carrot to move you forward and a stick to run away from. Why do you have to lose weight? What can you do to lose weight? Once committed, immediately do something toward the outcome of this commitment.

Dewey thinks about these questions and feels reluctant about the commitment. He does not want to fail but decides to try anyway.

A commitment I won't let myself back out of, with action? How do I do that? I'm not sure about this. I've failed many times, but I'd like to get my health in order and get away from that stick. I know I can change my diet to lose weight. The action I will take? I'll keep on this road and see what it has to offer.

Truly comes to the top of a hill, and thinks about how she lost weight with this new diet:

It feels good to have lost some weight, but this diet's restricting. It's, 'don't eat this' and 'stay away from that'. All I can think about is what I can't have, and that makes this harder. But, I have lost weight. So, I'll stick with it and lose more before the wedding.

Dewey walks up the path, and as it steepens, he comes upon a sign about an attitude check.

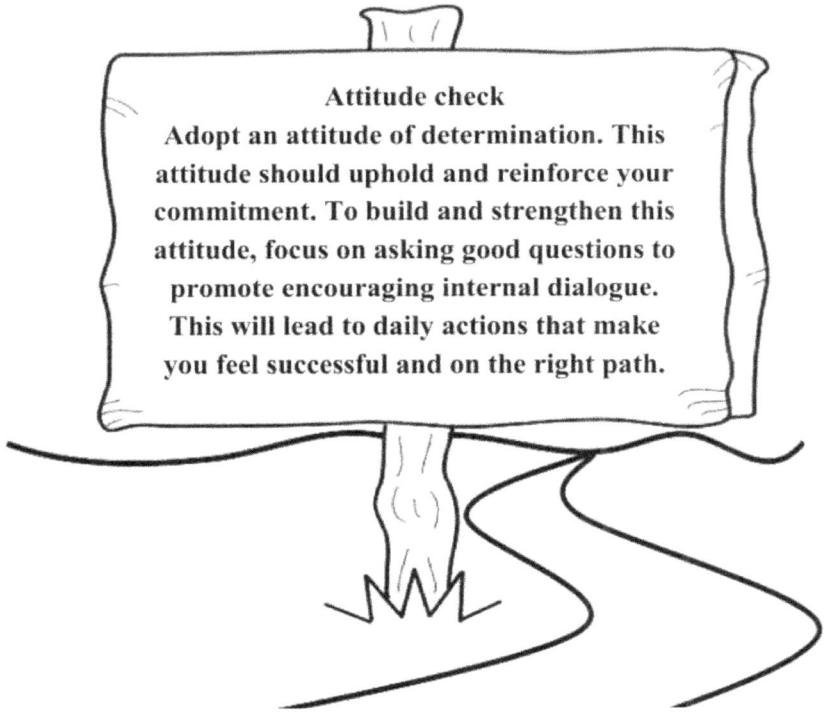

Attitude check

Adopt an attitude of determination. This attitude should uphold and reinforce your commitment. To build and strengthen this attitude, focus on asking good questions to promote encouraging internal dialogue. This will lead to daily actions that make you feel successful and on the right path.

Dewey reads the sign and begins working through the pitfalls of his attitude. He finds the questions he asks himself are not encouraging and the commitment he made is soft with a way out.

My commitment is not strong enough. I have serious health problems I have to fix, and losing weight is the first step to fixing them. I will lose weight, and I believe I can if I take action. The action I will take, no soda for one year. I hope the diet isn't too restricting.

Truly comes upon a speed bump and almost trips over a stick. She feels good to have lost some weight but is having trouble keeping to the new diet and begins secretly snacking late at night. Truly thinks about dieting and loses the momentum she had when she started this new diet.

It's hard to diet. It feels like I am trying to force my body to lose weight. I'm not sure about this, New Diet.

Dewey, heading up the long path, fully committed to his journey, sees the path level out a little after the starting line.

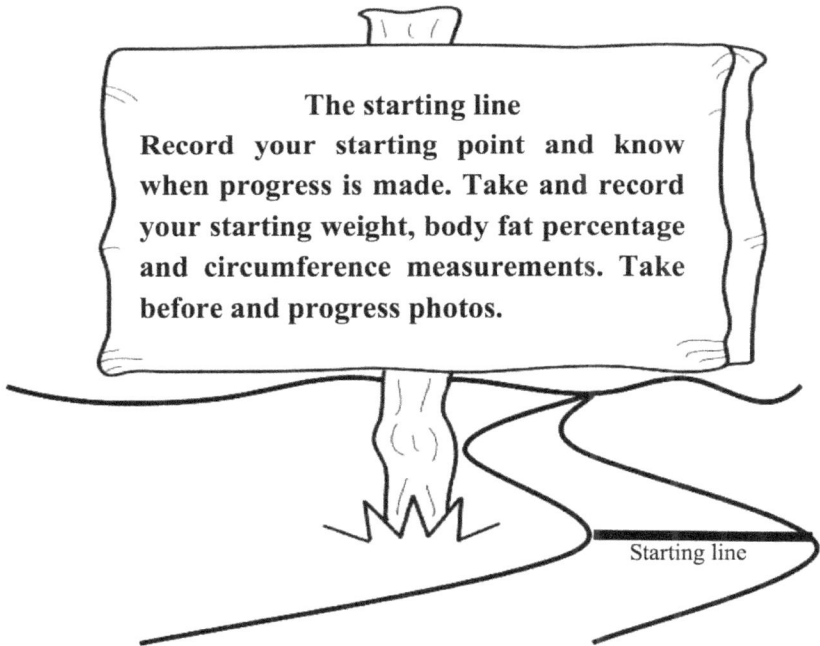

The starting line
Record your starting point and know when progress is made. Take and record your starting weight, body fat percentage and circumference measurements. Take before and progress photos.

Starting line

Dewey comes to the starting line and feels vulnerable at this moment. He reluctantly grabs a measuring tape, scale (that measures body fat, via bioimpedance), and camera. Privately recording the information, he thinks:

I can't believe I am doing this. Once I have my starting information, I will know if this path will produce results. I'm very curious about this path's diet. I hope I can still enjoy the food I eat.

Truly, discouraged by the speed bump and sticks just lying about, thinks:

This new diet isn't for me.

Once that thought passes through her mind, she sees a big piece of swiss cheese sitting on the side of the road and thinks:

Well, just a taste. A little bit won't hurt.

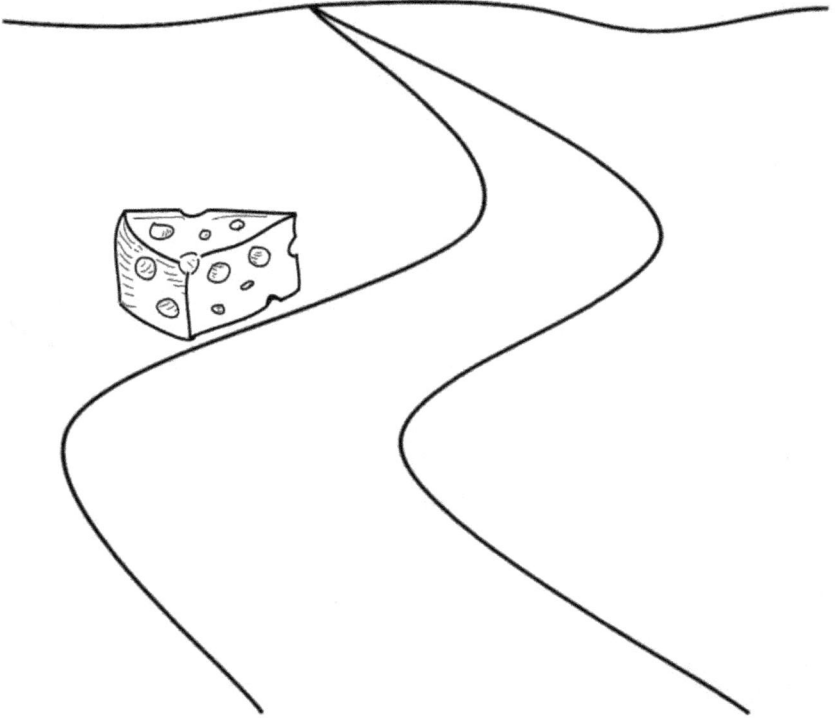

Dewey, curious about the diet, can't see where this path is going. He finds this sign about fueling the body.

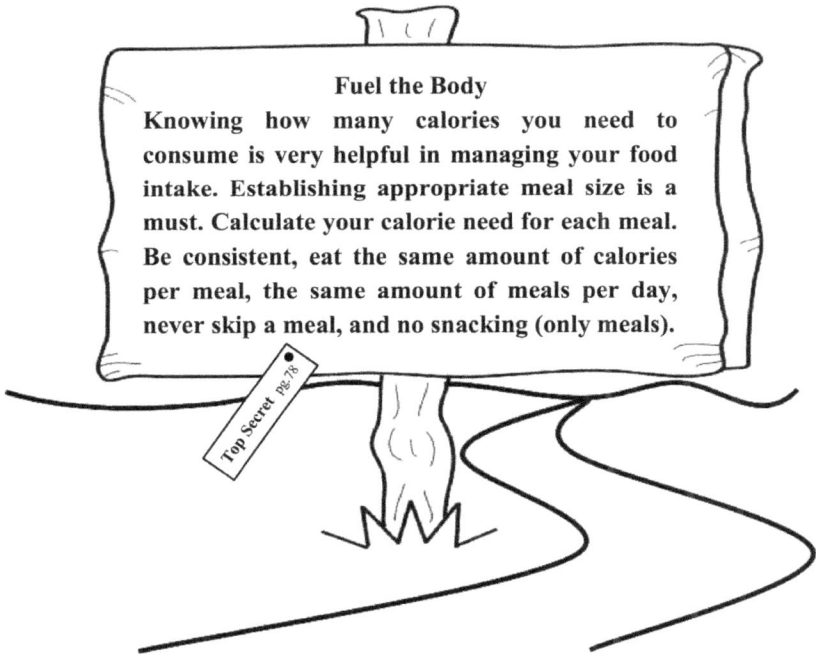

Fuel the Body

Knowing how many calories you need to consume is very helpful in managing your food intake. Establishing appropriate meal size is a must. Calculate your calorie need for each meal. Be consistent, eat the same amount of calories per meal, the same amount of meals per day, never skip a meal, and no snacking (only meals).

Dewey grabs and opens the envelope labeled, Top Secret. In the envelope, he learns how to calculate his calorie needs. He then thinks:

Ok, this is not the diet, but knowing how much to eat, will be helpful. Keeping my meals consistent with their calorie amount is an easy way to control portions. Over time, I'll learn how much I can eat of any meal. I can eat my favorite meals, as long as my portion size fits my 'per meal' calorie goal? There's got to be more to this.

Truly descends into a valley as she finishes the cheese. She sits on the side of the road and looks at the crumbs on her lap. Feeling the weight of regret and uncomfortable with her current state of mind, she uses a little humor to help push her forward.

Welp that didn't work. I wonder what other kinds of cheeses this road has to offer.

In a show of strength she says out loud:
"I need to get serious, the wedding is getting closer, and I want to lose some of this weight."

Dewey, heading up the path, sees a series of signs. Feeling overwhelmed, his eye widen as he imagines what the signs might say.

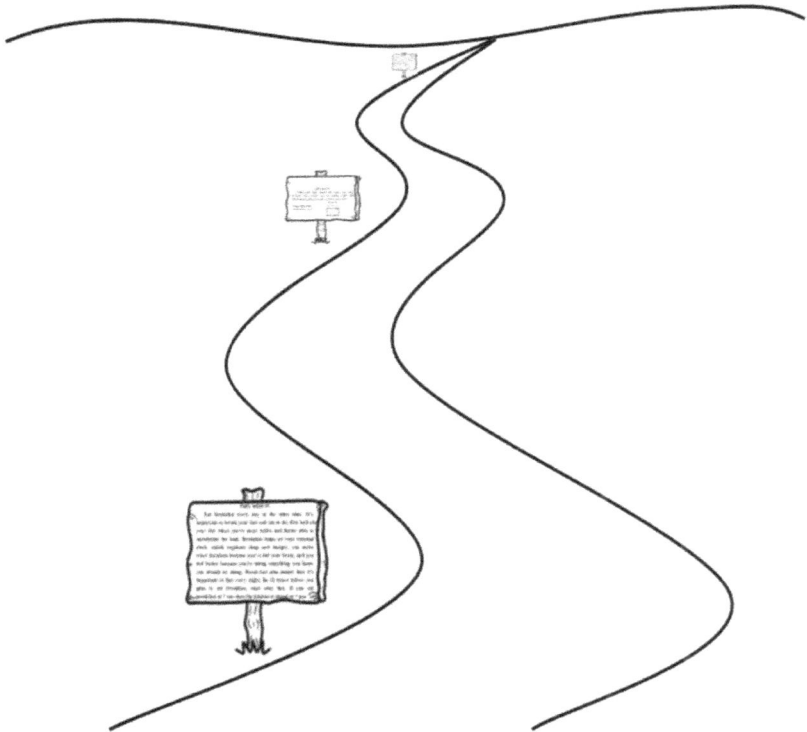

Daily Habit #1

Eat breakfast every day at the same time and set a daily eating routine. It is important to break your fast and eat in the first half of your day because you are more active and better able to metabolize the food. Breakfast helps to set your internal clock, which regulates sleep and hunger and you will make wiser decisions because you have fed your brain. Break-fast means it is important to fast every night. 12 hours before you plan to eat breakfast, start your fast. Example: breakfast is eaten at 7 am, close the kitchen at 7 pm.

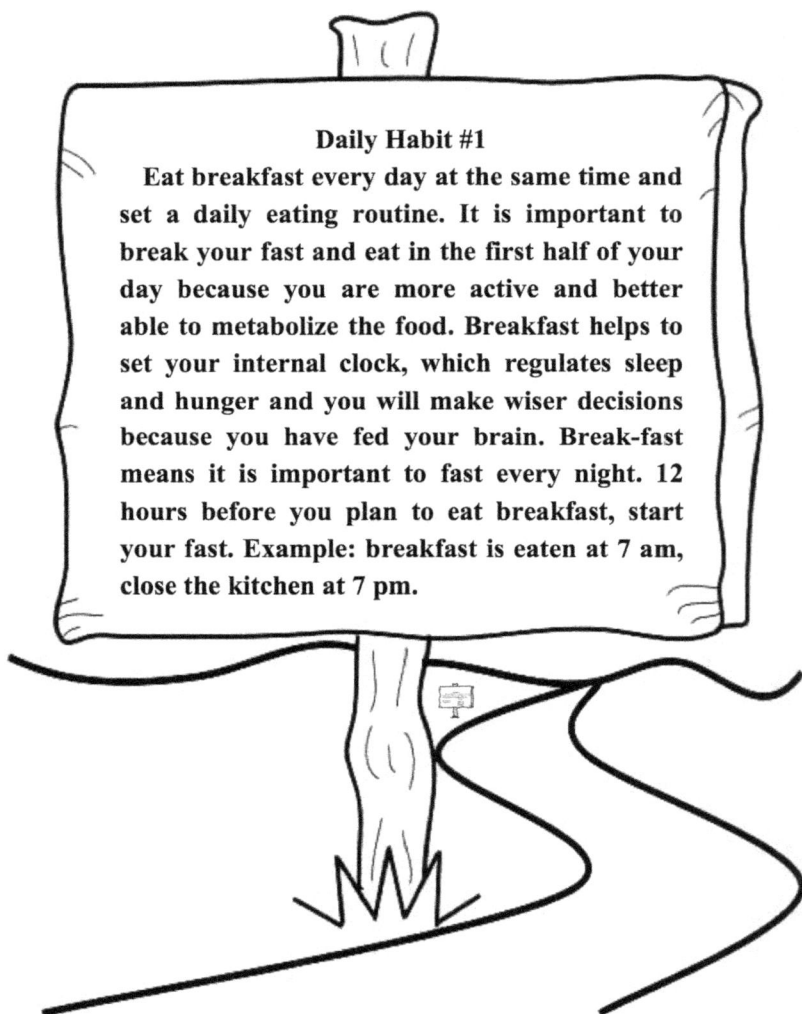

After reading the sign, he sees another sign ahead.

Daily Habit #2
Make good food choices, eat complete
meals and keep your body hydrated. Stay
focused, eat healthy foods with minimum
processing and drink mostly or only water.
Take One

-Eating suggestions.
-What should I eat?

Eating Suggestions.
What should I eat?

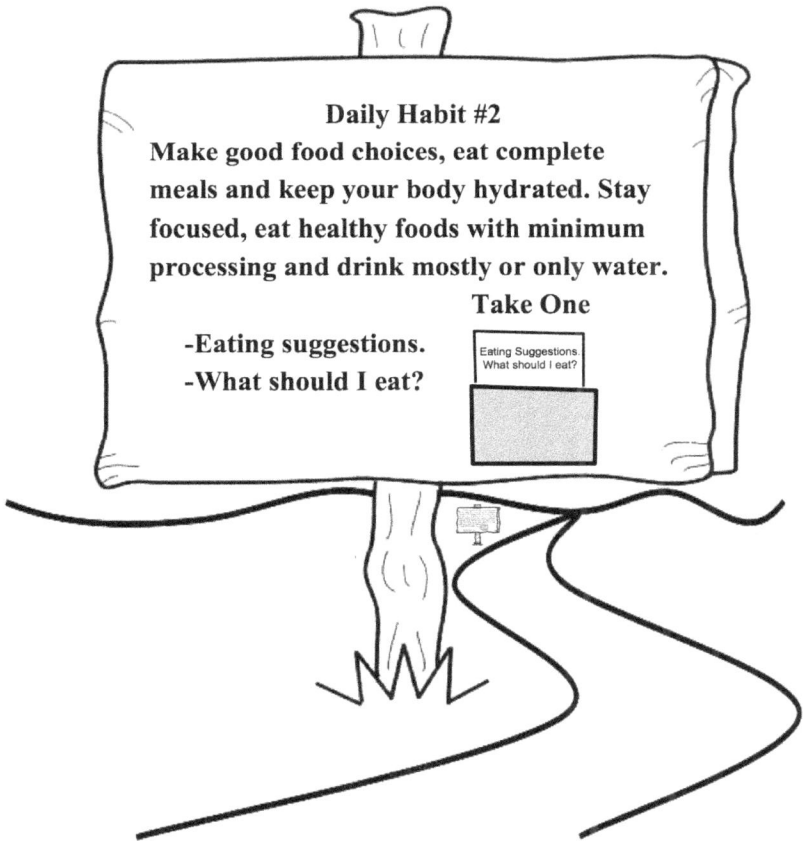

Dewey reads the sign and sees a pamphlet attached. He grabs one and reads it.

Eating suggestions.

- Trust your instincts. If you think, *I shouldn't eat this*, take the opportunity to make a better choice.
- Be consistent. Eat the same amount of calories in each meal and the same amount of meals in a day.
- A meal consists of protein, carbs, fats, and fiber.
- No snacking. Instead, create small 100 calorie meals. Each meal with protein, fats, carbs, and fiber.
- Educate yourself. Learn what 100 calories looks like of common foods you eat.
- Drink mostly water. Include coffee and tea with minimal to no additives.
- Increase the number of non-starchy vegetables you are eating. Hungry? Eat some veggies.
- Create a diet that fits your needs. Start by finding two breakfasts, two lunches and two dinners that meet your, per meal, calorie need. Build a meal base by adding two breakfasts, two lunches and two dinners each week for 6 weeks to your kitchen's menu.
- Enjoy the food you eat. Choose healthy foods you could enjoy for a lifetime. Take the food you already enjoy and turn these foods into healthy meals.
- Eat slowly. This helps you taste and enjoy your food, aids digestion, and lets you feel when you are full.
- It may prove helpful to avoid problem foods until you can introduce them to a healthy diet.

What should I eat?

- A plant-rich diet. Include plants in every meal.
- Eat a high protein breakfast.
- Eat naturally found, whole foods with minimum processing. Let your body do the processing, it's truly helpful. When we eat highly processed foods (like white flour, high fructose corn syrup, and partially hydrogenated oils) we send our hormones out of balance, making it difficult to utilize body fat for energy needs.
- Eat your veggies and eat them often. (1 cup is approximately 100 calories) Vegetables are very nutrient dense and do not pack a lot of calories. Eat onions, shallots, celery, carrots, tomato, garlic, corn, artichoke, squash, ginger, peas, lemongrass, leek, zucchini, brussels sprouts, eggplant, broccoli, cauliflower, bell pepper, asparagus, mushroom, lettuce, chives, peppers, spinach, scallions, kale, green beans, cabbage, jicama, cucumbers, etc.
- Eat whole fruits. (1 cup is approximately 100 calories) Fruits are very nutritious and packed with life. Eat an apple, orange, banana, tangerine, kiwi, peach, pear, plum, strawberry, blueberry, blackberry, raspberry, lemon, lime, etc.
- Eat the rainbow. (Blue, Green, Red, Orange, Yellow, Purple) We get vitamins and protective enzymes from the colorful pigments in food.

- Eat raw, unprocessed foods daily. Make one of your meals all raw foods or add a raw food item to your meal. Salads work.
- Eat fiber-rich carbohydrates (½ cup is about 100 calories) like beans, legumes, 100% whole grain or quinoa pastas, 100% whole grain breads (heavy in weight, rye or fermented sourdough bread where the yeast has been consuming the starches) oats, lentils, peas, corn, quinoa, brown and wild rice, sweet potatoes, yams, etc. Fiber is inside and in the skins of many different grains, fruits, and vegetables. Eat fiber daily, and everything will flow smoothly. Introduce fiber into your diet slowly.
- Eat healthy forms of fat (1 tablespoon is about 100 calories). Include extra virgin olive oil, avocado oil, canola oil and ghee. Also eat fats from avocados, nuts, seeds, and fish. Eating healthy fats will help you lose weight, aid digestion and the absorption of certain vitamins (A, D, E & K).
- Eat protein from beans, rice, legumes, nuts, tofu, quinoa, soy, wheat, corn, dairy, and animal meats.
- Choose good sources of dairy products or substitute with an organic soy or nut variety.

- Eat lean portions of animal meats (2 oz is about 100 calories). Eat fish like Cod, Sole, Salmon, Shrimp, Halibut, Tilapia, Rock Fish and land animals, like lean Chicken and Turkey, lean Beef and Pork.
- Use animal products to please the taste buds, to add substance and satiety to your meal and as a centerpiece to bring people together. Eating complete proteins are helpful in building body tissues like muscle, hormones and brain matter.
- Drink mostly water. Love your water. It will love you back. Drinking mostly water helps to eliminate unnecessary calories, and a dehydrated body finds it difficult to use stored body fat. Keeping hydrated also helps to rid the body of minor ailments and therefore, helps to ease the body through changes. Drinking water regularly plays many other functions including the removal of toxins, cushioning the joints, transporting oxygen and nutrients and helps your metabolism work properly, all of which help in the reduction of body fat.
- Flavor your food with salt, pepper, herbs, and spices. Find or make quality dry rubs and marinades.

Dewey reads about what he should eat and the eating suggestions and thinks:

The diet isn't "a diet" it's choosing to eat healthily and to find meals that meet my, per meal, calorie goal. I knew there was more to it. The part I like about this diet, I can lose weight using any dietary method, from a vegan diet to a meat lovers diet and everything in between, I will choose good ingredients and keep my portions under control. It looks like I got a little bit of homework to do for the next few weeks.

Dewey comes upon a clearing and sees the mountain this path is leading him up. He looks at the mountain, thinks about the homework and then remembers why he started this journey.

I have to get away from this stick. My doctor says my health problems will not go away until I lose weight and I know I need to eat a healthier diet. What I am going to do is create a healthy diet I can enjoy for a lifetime.

Seeing another sign up ahead, he runs to see what it says.

Daily Habit #3

Exercise often to build your metabolism. Focus on burning more calories than you consume, not consuming fewer calories than you burn. You can either make time to exercise or let time make you. Working out first thing in the morning will rev up your metabolism and help you to burn more fat throughout your day. Regular intense exercise burns calories and helps to improve carbohydrate metabolism and overall well being.

Find fun activities to keep you moving.

Take one
-Reasons to exercise
-Exercise guidelines

-Reasons to exercise
-Exercise guidelines

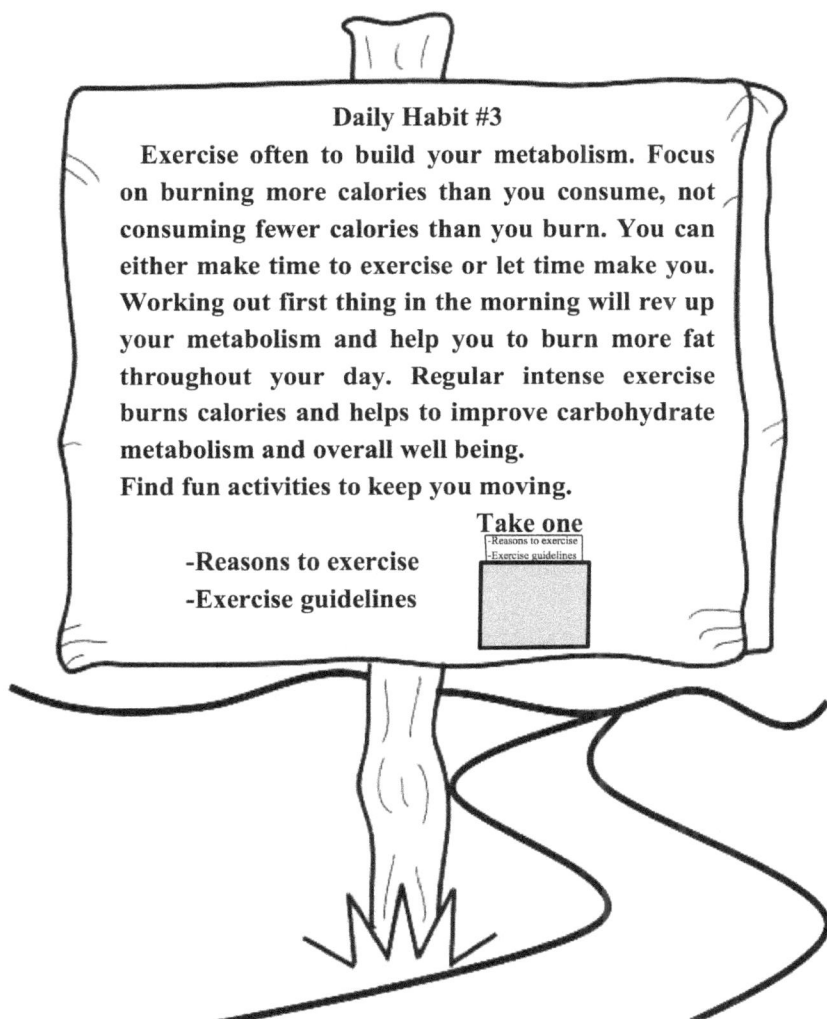

Duey reads the sign and sees there is another pamphlet attached, he grabs one and reads it.

Reasons to exercise

- Exercising helps every area of your life.
- Exercise improves mental and physical health.
- Exercise helps to ease daily stress, which improves your quality of life, and it will help you age gracefully.
- Exercising burns calories, strengthens your immune system, improves circulation, and the absorption of oxygen and nutrients. All important for life, weight loss and general well being.
- Being physically active in your life will help you manage carbohydrates. When you exercise regularly, you will improve and regulate carbohydrate metabolism and 12 to 16 hours after exercise, your body will be recovering and will have a higher metabolic rate. i.e., you'll burn more calories throughout your day.
- Exercising improves your heart and lungs. Getting your heart rate up provides oxygen to your working muscles and strengthens your ability to absorb oxygen into your bloodstream. Pay attention to and be a better breather, because we utilize fat for energy in an aerobic state (aerobic metabolism).
- Exercise strengthens your muscles. Muscle is metabolic tissue. The more muscle you have, the more calories you'll burn. If you don't use your muscles (strength training), you'll lose your muscles (muscle atrophy).

- Overload your muscles with resistance. It helps prevent muscle loss, increases muscle mass, and improves your metabolism. How often do you flex and exhaust your muscles?
- The impact that occurs during exercise makes bone denser and builds a stronger body frame.
- Exercise is one of the best stress management tools you got. If you want to lose weight and keep it off, you must deal with stress productively. Also, regular exercise increases self-confidence.
- Exercise tires the body, so you get a good night's sleep. Tire the body, quiet the mind, and sleep soundly.
- Exercising sends an abundance of freshly oxygenated blood to your oxygen thirsty brain, and you need to supply your brain with what it needs to make these changes permanent.
- Exercising helps to create a positive attitude towards life. Your attitude determines: where you go, how long it takes and how easy it is for you to get there. When you exercise regularly, you feel better and thus a better attitude because you are accomplishing something hard on a regular basis.
- Exercising should not feel like a chore. If it does, then choose another form of exercise.

Exercise Guidelines

- Find healthy activities to grow in your journey.
- Focus on the F.B.I. (form, breath, intensity). It will turn any activity into an exercise session. <u>Form</u> (head up, shoulders back and down, belly button in). <u>Breath deeply</u> (in through the nose, press the air out or four breaths in, then four breaths out). <u>Intensity</u> (increase intensity to raise your metabolic rate and burn more calories during and after exercise).
- Get your heart rate up every day and provide oxygen to your brain and working muscles.
- The objective, in the beginning, is to set a schedule and get into a good routine. As you become more comfortable with exercising, you want to add other types of exercise and gradually increase your intensity while always controlling breath and form.
- Always warm-up and cool-down. This initial low intensity, deep breathing, good form exercise help to stretch veins and arteries and prepare your body for exercise. This low intensity, full breath exercise uses an abundance of fat energy in your working muscles. After a good warm-up, increase your intensity and get your heart rate up. Then gradually lower the intensity. Now for the cool-down. This low-intensity activity

brings the body back from intense exercise and promotes the healing of stressed or damaged tissues.

- Start all new exercise activities on easy mode and build your ability to tolerate higher intensity exercises. Be wise and keep intensity low for the first few weeks.
- Strengthen your muscles. You strengthen your muscles by overloading them with resistance (leveraging body weight is all you need). When losing weight, strength training is about maintaining your muscle mass and increasing your metabolism. After you lose weight turn your focus to building muscle (the secret to keeping the weight off).
- Do intense fitness training two to three days a week. Intense training is predetermined periods of higher intensity training. Intense training is hard it's pushing yourself outside of your comfort zone. Include strength and cardio exercises.
- Stretch or do yoga. Spend 10 minutes stretching daily or take a yoga class 1 day a week. Focus on the F.B.I. of exercise, during stretching and yoga sessions. Stretching helps prevent injuries and promotes good energy flow in the body.

Truly's pace slows as the road gets windy. Suddenly, around a sharp turn, she trips on a stick, and it flips up and hits her. She rubs her leg as she reads a sign that suggests a weight loss supplement.

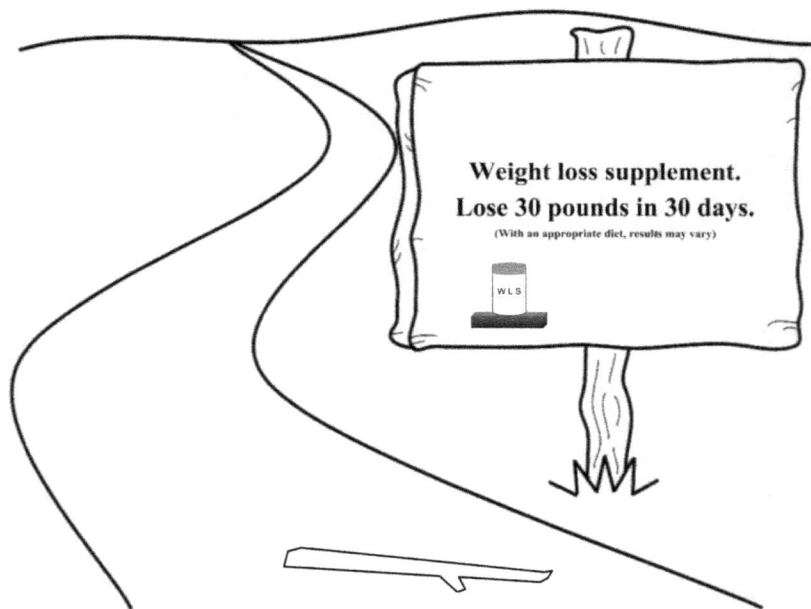

Weight loss supplement.
Lose 30 pounds in 30 days.
(With an appropriate diet, results may vary)

WLS

Truly reads the sign and thinks:
Lose 30 pounds in 30 days, that's perfect. A supplement to help me lose weight, before the wedding.
She grabs the suppliment and starts taking it.

Dewey, heading up a mountain, sees a sign about behavior change.

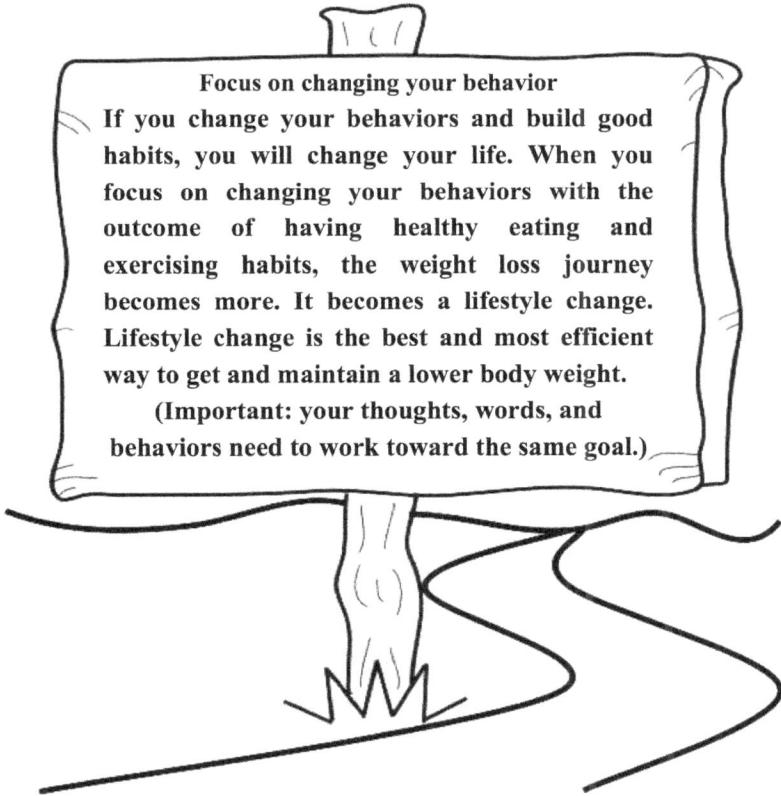

Focus on changing your behavior

If you change your behaviors and build good habits, you will change your life. When you focus on changing your behaviors with the outcome of having healthy eating and exercising habits, the weight loss journey becomes more. It becomes a lifestyle change. Lifestyle change is the best and most efficient way to get and maintain a lower body weight.

(Important: your thoughts, words, and behaviors need to work toward the same goal.)

Dewey looks at his behaviors and thinks:

If I focus on changing my behaviors around food and exercise, I will begin to build a healthy lifestyle. This lifestyle will help me lose weight. Once I get to my ideal weight, the same lifestyle is how I maintain it. Behaviors are something in my control and my behavior around exercising needs a little work.

He decides to pick up the pace and starts jogging.

Truly, noticing the well-traveled road getting a little rough, and the wedding looming ever closer. She was able to lose a few pounds but doesn't like how this supplement is making her feel.

I feel weird, antsy and jittery, ever since I've been taking this supplement, but it did work. The wedding is tomorrow, and I am glad I was able to lose some weight. Not as much as I wanted, but it will have to do.

Dewey is jogging steadily on the smooth path. He comes upon a sign about finding a fitness goal.

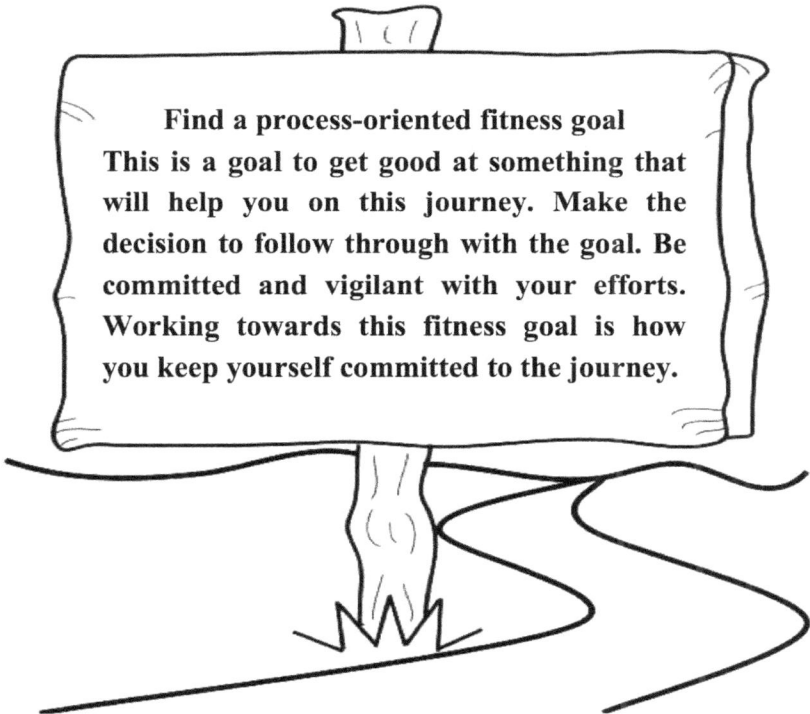

Find a process-oriented fitness goal
This is a goal to get good at something that will help you on this journey. Make the decision to follow through with the goal. Be committed and vigilant with your efforts. Working towards this fitness goal is how you keep yourself committed to the journey.

Dewey reads the sign and thinks:
So this is how I keep myself committed to this process. I need to get leverage on myself and find a process goal (carrot) that moves me away from my health problems (stick). My carrot will be to get good at cooking healthy food. I've always wanted to learn how to cook, and this is the best time to learn. I can't wait to have delicious, healthy meals I know how to cook well. I will become a good cook. For the first time, I know I can do this.

Truly's road is a little rough with loose gravel and lots of potholes, she lost some weight with the supplement and had a good time at the wedding. But after she stopped taking the supplement, she started gaining the weight back.

"This is impossible. I'll never lose this weight and keep it off."

Sitting slowly on to the curb, looking at her belly. She closes her eyes, slumps her shoulders and sighs, deep in thought...

Dewey's path smooths out and gets easier to travel. Jogging up the path, he finds a sign and starts putting it all together.

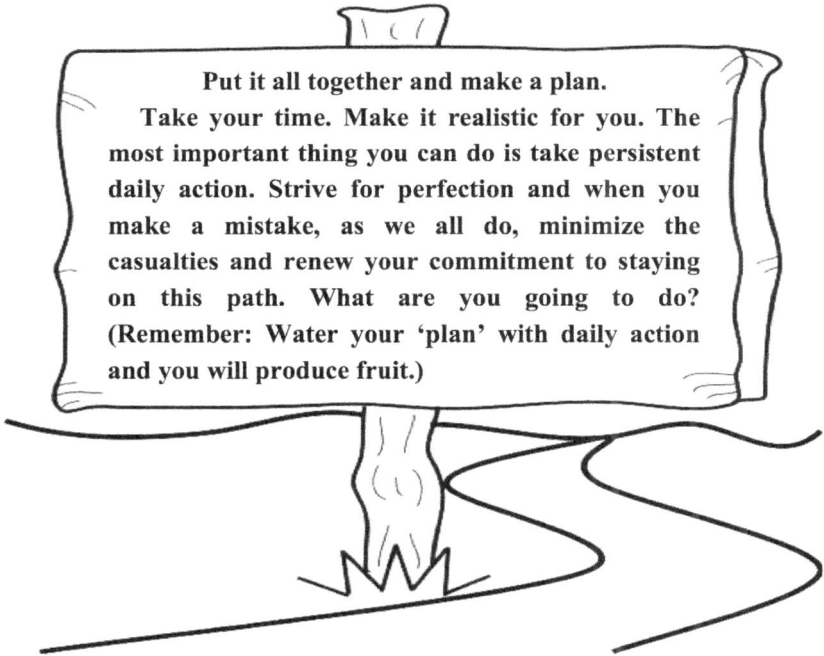

> **Put it all together and make a plan.**
> Take your time. Make it realistic for you. The most important thing you can do is take persistent daily action. Strive for perfection and when you make a mistake, as we all do, minimize the casualties and renew your commitment to staying on this path. What are you going to do? (Remember: Water your 'plan' with daily action and you will produce fruit.)

After thinking about what he is going to do, he starts developing a plan.

I will learn how to cook healthy food and water my plan with daily action. My plan, to build the habit of eating breakfast, keep my calories under control by finding meals that fit my calorie needs and make time to exercise. I will be able to build off this plan.

Feeling excited about his goal, he sees the path that will lead him to hear those words 'I did it'.

Truly feels beat up from the rough road, and thinks about her failures as the road she travels twists and turns. She finds a little hope when she sees a sign that guarantees her weight loss.

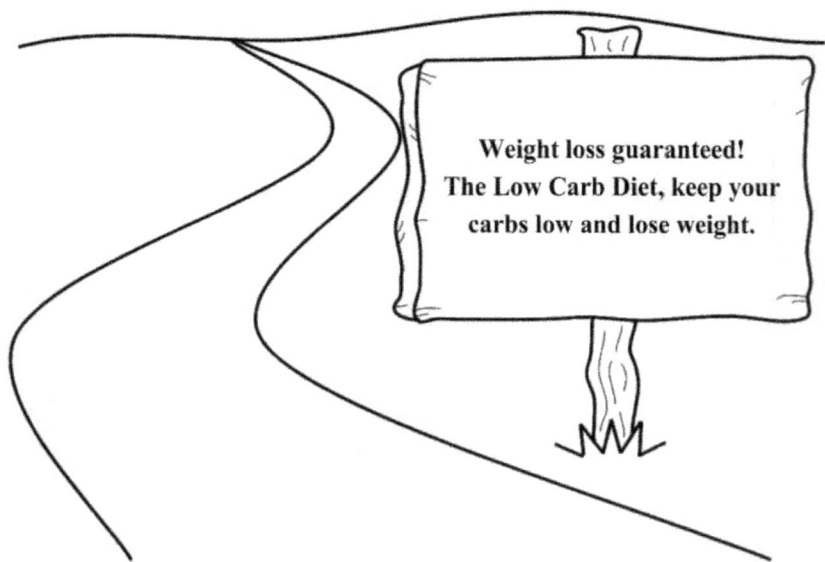

**Weight loss guaranteed!
The Low Carb Diet, keep your
carbs low and lose weight.**

She reads the sign and thinks:

I've heard I can lose weight on this diet. I will try this diet, lose weight and keep it off.

Dewey travels steadily up the mountain as he puts his plan to work. After a few months of losing weight, he thinks:

My commitment to this process goal has been the cornerstone of my success. I am becoming a good cook. I have found quite a few delicious meals that I cook very well. I make sure to drink enough fresh water and put the eating and exercising suggestions to work. I eat a plant-rich diet full of non-starchy vegetables, whole fruits, healthy fats and lean meat and fish. There was a lot of highly processed corn and wheat in my diet, it was worth keeping these to a minimum. It took time to find healthy meals I enjoy and meet my per meal calorie needs but learning how to cook has proven to be a valuable skill in this part of the journey. I developed a good routine of what I eat, and when I eat it and I'm well on my way to having healthy eating habits. I jog most mornings and follow that with a high protein breakfast. This process is working I can see this being something I do for a long time. I found it difficult to get started but simple and effective once I got going.

Truly travels to new heights on her road and it put her in a good mood because she has been losing weight. Her clothes are now a little too big, so she went and bought all new clothes.

I have been watching the scale go down, and that's great, but this diet makes me feel a little weak. I haven't had much energy lately, it would be hard to do this for a long time. I think I will add a cheat day, so I'm not suffering all the time. It feels great to lose weight, but I can't wait until I can eat more carbs. This diet works, I look good in my new clothes. I will hold onto my old clothes, just in case.

Dewey hit a speed bump on the path while putting his plan through the life test. He thinks about how he initially lost a lot of weight, but the weight loss seems to have stopped.

I haven't lost much weight lately, but I feel great. I have been sleeping better, and my doctor says that my health has improved and to keep doing what I've been doing. I'm getting away from the health problem stick that was hitting me. My focus is on building healthy eating habits because I want to see if the habit will make the food part easier. My morning jog has been good, but once I committed to it, it got easier to enjoy it. Getting my blood pumping early in the day, it wakes me up and gives me some personal, alone time before the craziness of my day. Now that I have lost some weight by building healthy eating and exercising habits, it's time to break through this plateau. I will re-calculate my calorie needs and add some intense fitness training. I can manage 30 minutes 3 days a week, and keep, my personal, jogging time in the morning.

Thinking about this journey and where he began, he cannot help but wonder how Truly has been doing, and if she has lost any weight.

Truly hit a speed bump in the road and has not been able to lose any more weight. Feeling frustrated after mostly losing the weight. She is eating more carbs than she should, to maintain the weight she lost.

I've done what I wanted to do and lost a lot of weight. I just want to lose a little more, but this last little bit will not come off. The cheat day has been helpful, at least I'm not torturing myself all the time. I should be able to eat a little more carbs, now that I have lost the weight.

Dewey, traveling steadily up the path, picks up his pace and adds intense fitness training. He thinks about how he broke through his plateau and lost more weight.

I started doing intense fitness training and broke through a plateau. I lost most of the weight I wanted to, then I added some strength training. I increase my muscle mass (my calorie burning ability), after six months, I feel good about where I am with my weight. I go for a jog every morning, eat breakfast every day and do intense exercise for 30 to 45 minutes, 3 to 4 days a week. I have a good routine and have ingrained this exercising habit. With my eating habit set, the food part is easier. There are times when I'm tempted by old ways, I turn that into an opportunity, rework my internal language and push through that moment. The healthy eating habit gave me a chance to take the focus off food, keep my food right because this is how I eat and focus on exercising (burning more calories than I consume). Now that I have the habit of, frequently exercising with intensity, I can adjust my exercise intensity, the amount of time I spend and the types of exercises I do, based on new goals.

Truly's road gets rocky as she gains some of the weight back. After eating a somewhat normal diet, she thinks:

I'm happy to have lost weight. The clothes I bought are getting a little tight, but that's ok. I still look good, and at least I'm not where I was.

Truly, reminiscing about all the good times thinks:

I've been having a good time hanging out with old friends. We've been going out dancing and enjoying happy hours. It reminds me of when I use to hang out with Dewey. I wonder what he's up to I haven't heard from him in a while.

Dewey makes it to the top of the mountain. He's lost the weight he carried most of his life.

I've worked hard to get healthy and lose weight. The first 6 weeks I did a lot of work, finding delicious, healthy meals and over time, I was able to create a healthy menu for my kitchen. I eat the right amount of calories per meal, and I exercise on a regular, consistent schedule. Making a plan helped keep me on this path, I knew what I was going to do because I already made the decision. I wasn't struggling, and that was a nice shift.

Dewey enjoying the views atop his mountain steps onto a scale and throws a fist in the air, yelling out loud,

"I did it I did it. The weight is finally gone."

He bought new clothes and made a few decisions.

I am committed to keeping this weight off, and I know I can because I love the lifestyle I created. I'm getting rid of all my old clothes because I will NEVER wear those again. Actually. I will keep one pair of jeans, just as a reminder. My new process goal (carrot) will be to get better at weightlifting. I will re-calculate my calorie needs and adjust my meals, to meet my new goal. This lifestyle will be a hobby of mine.

Truly falls back into her old ways, and her road drops quickly into a deep valley. She's gained the weight back plus a few pounds. Truly looks down at the road while she drags her feet deep in thought. She stops, looks up and says in a sad tone.

"I have tried and tried and I still can't seem to get rid of this weight. I lose weight, only to gain it back again. I give up, let's face it, I'm always going to be fat."

Dewey on his mountaintop begins thinking:
Is this all there is.

He decides to keep moving along this path and suddenly ran into an important sign that says to pay it forward.

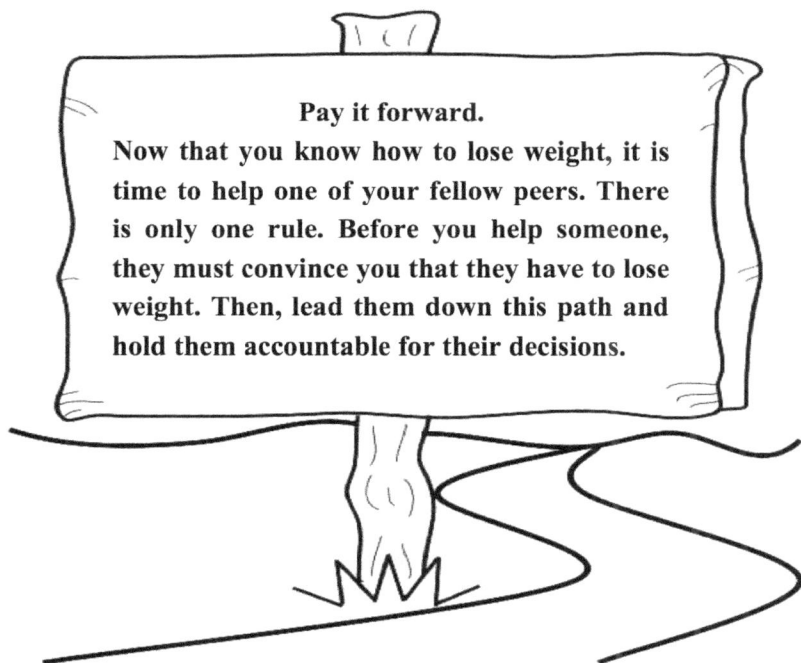

Pay it forward.
Now that you know how to lose weight, it is time to help one of your fellow peers. There is only one rule. Before you help someone, they must convince you that they have to lose weight. Then, lead them down this path and hold them accountable for their decisions.

Pay it forward by helping somebody take this path. I get to help someone and ingrain this lifestyle at the same time. I am going to do this. Where do I find somebody in need of guidance? I know, I will go back to where I started and find someone ready to change.

Truly, hanging her head low in failure, finds the end of the road.

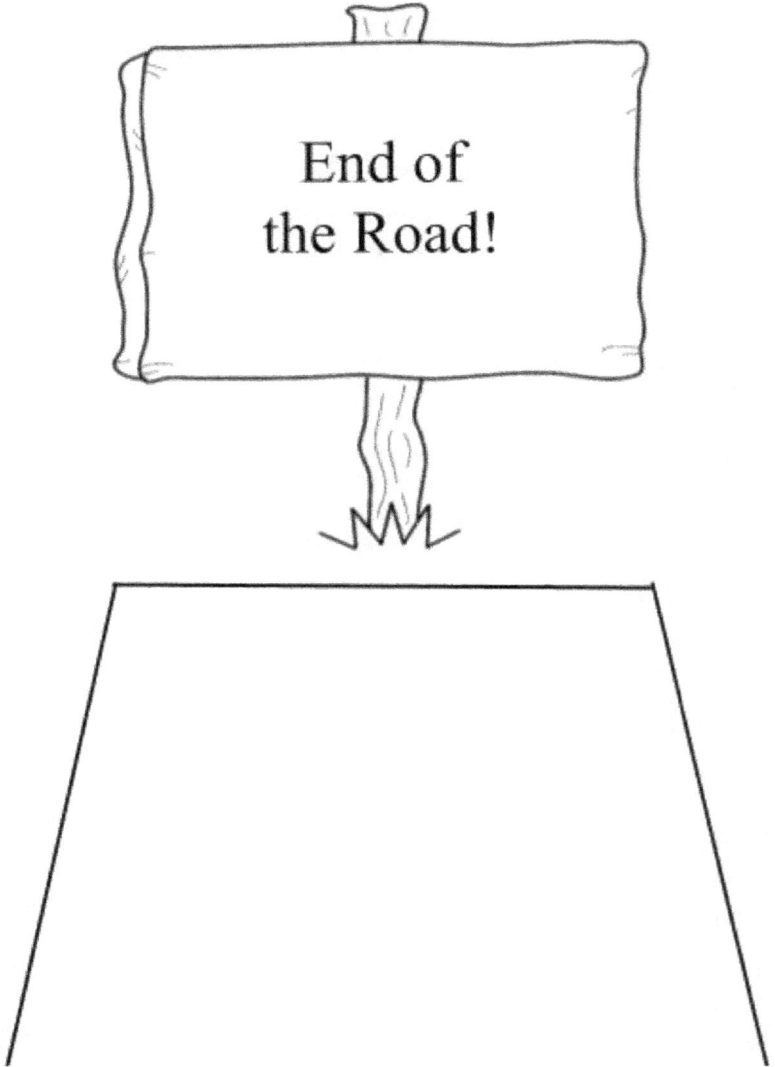

End of
the Road!

Truly, with all her frustrations, stumble on the rocky bottom at the end of the road and thinks:

I'm tired of being fat and always fighting an uphill battle. Losing weight, to gain it back has got to stop. I will do whatever it takes but what do I need to do? Where do I begin? How do I keep the weight off once I have lost it?

Truly finds strength and says out loud:

"Please, can someone help me!"

Dewey sets out on his journey to find a friend in need of guidance. On his way, he runs into his old friend Truly.

"Hey Truly, how are you?"

"Fine, I guess. Wow, Dewey, you look great. How did you lose the weight? I have been trying and trying, and the weight won't stay off."

"Have you been trying to lose weight since the last time I saw you?"

"Yes, I lost weight for that wedding, then I tried again and lost a lot of weight, but I keep gaining it back. You lost weight, how did you do it?"

"Good, I like the questions. Before we get to that, why do you have to lose weight?"

"Why do I have to lose weight? Isn't it obvious? Are you willing to help me or not."

"Yes Truly, I am willing to help. But, I have to make sure you need to change. So before I can help you, you must convince me that you are committed to making some life changes. Why do you have to lose weight?"

"You want me to convince you I have to lose weight? Waite isn't that what your friend Olive had you do. Ok, the reason I have to lose weight? I want to look in the mirror and like what I see. I want to eat without wondering if I'm going to gain weight."

Truly's eyes get heavy with tears,

"I need to take control of my health and set a good example for my kids. I don't want them to end up in this situation. I am fed up with being overweight and feeling like a failure, out of control and helpless in my own body. I need to break the cycle of losing weight only to gain it back."

With a renewed sense of strength.

"This stuff has gone on long enough, and it has to change, and it is going to change, whether you help me or not. Am I committed enough for you."

"Yes Truly, I can feel your commitment, and I can see you are already on the right path. Losing weight affects many areas of our lives, and it's hard to hold onto a new you, without a spoken commitment to yourself and the people around you. It's time, you're ready and now let me show you the right path."

Dewey shows Truly the path he took, and she starts to develop her plan.

"Ok, Dewey. I'm getting it. The most important thing is to get leverage on myself, take daily action towards my carrot and/or run away from the stick that keeps hitting me. My kids are learning my bad habits, and that has to change, I will run as fast as I can from that stick. I am committed to be consistent and eat my calorie goal (breakfast, lunch, and dinner), go for a walk every day, and fast (12 hours) between dinner and breakfast. I am committed to eating a plant-rich diet full of non-starchy vegetables and to drink plenty of fresh water. I like this plan it allows me to start losing weight while I find healthy meals and develop healthy eating habits. My process goal, or carrot, will be to get better at running. I have always wanted to run a marathon and will do it next fall. I believe I can do this."

"That's what I wanted to hear, and I know you can," Dewey said. "If you believe in yourself and find a process goal you want to achieve, this mountain will feel more manageable to climb. Now that I know what you are committed to doing, I can help keep your standards up and push you to be your best. Without this commitment, my help would be useless because ultimately you have to do the work. I will give you some tips I learned to help you through this process."

"Thank you." Truly said.

Truly put her plan to work, and after many months of climbing the mountain, she achieved her goal. Shes worked to be a better runner and ran a marathon. She found her confidence and knows how to keep the weight off. Truly tells Dewey about what she learned from this process.

"I know how to lose weight, and keep it off. I choose to eat appropriate meal sizes using minimally processed nutritious ingredients and keep my body strong and active. I struggled with letting go of old habits, and I had emotional issues I had to deal with, but once I did, I began to enjoy a new lifestyle, and the road smoothed out for me. I also found a good support group that helped get me through rough roads and I'm being careful not to create hard moments through the negative, repetitive self-talk I sometimes do. When the weight loss slowed, and my body started to balance itself out, I increased my workout intensity and started doing new types of exercises."

"It sounds like you are doing it right, Truly."

Dewey and Truly worked hard, and both lost their extra weight. They discuss this process of losing weight and had this to say.

"Losing weight is hard." Truly said. "It affected areas of my life I didn't expect. If I want to lose weight for an event or get the ball rolling, a quick diet change would help me do that, but if I want to keep the weight off, my lifestyle had to change. I think that's the hardest part because it changed my family life, outings with friends and how I deal with stress. There isn't a quick fix for a long time problem, it's a process, and it takes time."

"I think your right Truly, it does take time. The hardest part for me was learning to enjoy this new lifestyle, finding meals and workouts I could get excited about. I immersed myself in the journey and developed a lifestyle that produced real results. I thought it was the results I liked, but the journey is what I enjoyed. I grew from every meal, every workout, I got stronger mentally, physically and emotionally. I was changing, and that scared me, I didn't know what to expect. I pushed through my fear, and the roots of my fitness foundation took hold. I was never going back."

"Alright Dewey, I need to pay it forward and find someone in need of guidance. You know, I am already paying it forward to my kids, that was the stick I was running away from. They have been learning by my example. They've seen how important it is to me and have shown interest in running while I was training for that marathon. I will continue to nurture this lifestyle through our living environment. I can influence them through my actions. When I see a genuine interest, I will encourage them towards a process goal."

"That's an awesome place to pay it forward I'm very proud of you Truly. You have come a long way."

Dewey and Truly have been learning how to lose weight for the past year and had a few insights they wanted to share.

You know what, Truly. After losing weight for the past year, I learned if I ate my per meal calorie goal and I made sure to exercise most days of the week, I was able to lose weight. With an improved diet and regular exercise, this journey turned into a lifestyle. I found changing your lifestyle is how you keep the weight off because if you go back to your old ways, you will gain the weight back like I have done many times before.

I agree with you, Dewey. We have to live an active, healthy lifestyle and burn more calories than we eat. The part I found fascinating is how this plan deals with carbohydrates. Instead of eliminating them, it uses them productively. I learned there are three ways this plan manages carbohydrates. The first way is by fasting for 12 hours every night (eating during the active part of your day), the second way by eating complete meals, and the third way is exercising regularly. These three practices help steady and lower circulating glucose and put you in a position where you'll use the readily available energy provided by carbohydrates for muscular activity. I also found that choosing to eat fiber-rich carbohydrates was also very helpful in this matter.

Truly settles into her life and decides she doesn't want to work out all the time, but she knows keeping the weight off is a matter of, give and take. She tells Dewey this is a lifelong journey she is going to travel.

"I have to condition the habit of eating a healthy diet until this is just how I eat, then condition some more. I will make cooking healthy food my process goal and get better at cooking. I may even write a cookbook. To keep active, I'll go on regular walks and enjoy fun activities (like dancing, softball, gardening or classes at the gym) to keep me active. I am committed to doing a certain amount of daily exercise to maintain and keep me healthy. I pledge to keep on this path of healthy eating and regular exercise. I will enjoy the natural shape of my body and learn to love who I am."

Dewey settles into his new life and found confidence with exercising. He became better at strength training and was able to gain a lot of muscle. He enjoys the freedom of being able to eat whatever he wants but still chooses to eat, whole, nutritious foods because he enjoys the fresh flavors and how these foods make him feel. He talks to Truly about the lifestyle he created,

"I found this lifestyle is much more than losing weight, although that was a benefit. It's about living healthy, so I age gracefully. I am going to eat healthily, exercise regularly, and live fully. This is my new life, and I love it."

The End
of the story.
Now is the time to
start your journey.

Dewey Do's Tips

Use them well.

Dewey Do's Tips

Put a check mark on the tips you will use.

☐**Always use your inner wisdom.** Listen to what your gut is telling you. Don't just follow someone's word blindly, find out if it is true and makes sense for you.

☐**Be flexible.** Find the program that best works for you, makes you feel empowered and successful.

☐**Get leverage on yourself.** Let's get real and find what will push you forward. Identify actions or non-actions that are holding you back. The carrot and the stick. How is the problem (stick) hurting you right now? How will, taking action towards a goal (carrot) benefit you now?

☐**Find your motivation.** Motivation is the reason that moves you towards what you want, and away from what you don't want. When you feel motivated, create momentum by taking action. When something happens, that halts your momentum, remember what motivates you. Keep on your path because if you have an "I will attitude" you will find your way.

☐**Get rid of your excuses**, especially the good ones. Excuses let you off the hook and keep you focused on the problem. Instead actively look to the solution. To be successful think, *how can I? What can I do?* Or, *this is why I like this!* Learn from experts and others who have been successful. You can also use your so-called failures as motivation to move you toward your goal.

□**It doesn't matter what happens in life.** What matters is how you feel about what happens. It's your choice.

□**Use the power of perspective.** Look at your situation from a different point of view it will change how you feel about your situation. This point of view will give you compassion and understanding, and make your struggles and challenges easier to overcome. Look at your attitude and actions through the eyes of another or a helicopter point of view and give yourself a new perspective on your situation. A new perspective can give you the edge you need to overcome your challenges. What you put your attention on is what is real to you at that moment. If you think, *"this sucks. I don't like this!"* Or *"Exercising sucks, I hate it!"* don't be surprised if those feelings intensify into reality.

□**Pay attention to your internal dialogue, and spoken language, it could be holding you back.** Be careful you may be talking yourself into making a mistake (rationalizing). Rework/re-word any inner dialogue that may be holding you back, so it moves you forward (talk yourself into eating healthy). Look for the "I can't," problem-finding type of thinking and begin to rework the language and engrain through repetition, a new internal dialogue. When you focus on what you like, you will find yourself secretly enjoying your journey. This sign says you're on the right path. Enjoyment is the foundation of lasting change and success.

☐**Stay out of your comfort zone.** You need to push yourself to stay focused. It's not always comfortable eating new types of foods, exhausting your muscles and managing stress. In fact, it's very uncomfortable to change our ways and adopt a new lifestyle. Be concerned if you feel comfortable in this journey.

☐**Set a bedtime and be in bed on time.** It helps you get the necessary sleep needed. When you're well rested, notice how much energy you have to burn. Body fat is where our bodies store excess energy.

☐**Educate yourself.** Education will help reinforce good habits. Good habits breed success.

☐**Meditate.** Meditation will lengthen your attention span and quiet the chatter in your mind, so you can listen to yourself and make wise decisions from that state of being (use your inner wisdom). Meditation is an exercise for the brain and is an exercise with extraordinary benefits. Search, find and then practice different meditation techniques. Still mind, reflect and analyze, listening to the body (heartbeat, breath, etc).

☐**Losing weight is not a forceful process.** It's difficult to force our bodies to lose weight we don't have that kind of control. You can influence your body to lose weight by getting your mind right (attitude, motivation), getting your food right (calories, food choice), and exercising in some form on a regular basis.

☐**Tell people around you.** Telling people around you puts social pressure on you. Use this pressure to your advantage. There's pressure because you've made a decision and now you have told someone. Be true to your word and take daily action when action is needed.

☐**Practice self-discipline.** Your words and actions must match. Remember nobody is perfect, we all make mistakes, and that's ok, mistakes are there to teach us if we quiet the chatter in our minds and listen. When we were little, some of us learned the hard way that the stove gets hot. We made a mistake, just don't let that mistake keep you from getting near the stove and learning how to cook.

☐**Surround yourself with good influences.** Find good food, encouraging people and activities you enjoy. Look at your environment, your home, car, workspace and see if it promotes the changes that you would like to make. Change what you can and don't put a lot of attention to the stuff you can't change.

☐**Recognize your successes.** Pat yourself on the back, tell yourself "good job" in a meaningful way. Be proud of your successes and tell people. Reward yourself with something not food related. Measure immediate success by your behavior (habits) and by your belt size. Use the scale as a tool for long-term success and to know when you've hit a milestone.

☐ **Ask Good questions.** Have a significant other, a friend, or hire a professional to ask good questions and keep you focused. Questions like: "How was your workout? What's for breakfast tomorrow? Are you going to work out tomorrow?"

☐ **Keep yourself focused and on task.** Create a collage. Put up pictures and create a visual goal. Write down reasons why you're doing this. Write inspirational and motivational quotes. Create a space to write stuff you've learned to be true. Read your collage every day to keep you on task.

☐ **Enjoy the process.** Focus on the journey (behavior and habit formation) and see consistent weight loss. We find happiness in the journey towards a goal. When you achieve a goal, you pass a milestone in life, and that feels good. But, true happiness is in the adventure towards the goal.

☐ **Belly laugh as much as possible.** Laughter feels good and is good for your mental health.

☐ **Keep your head up.** Literally, keep your head up. Having good posture (head up, shoulders back and down) will promote a good attitude, you feel the way you think and hold your body. Hold yourself like a depressed person does (body language, facial expression, and mental thought), and you'll feel down or depressed. The opposite is also true if you sit up, smile, and think optimistically you will feel a little better. You'll notice it takes work to hold your body with good posture and work equals used calories.

☐**Make sure you have comfortable shoes.**

☐**Flex and Exhaust your muscles.** A body that flexes and exhausts its muscles daily will burn more calories throughout the day because of the recent workout session. After a workout our bodies have a higher metabolic rate, meaning you'll burn calories at a higher rate after the workout. There's also a compounding effect that takes place. Flexing and exhausting your muscles will strengthen and build muscle, your ability to burn calories. The more muscle you have, the more calories you'll burn. Flexing and exhausting your muscles during weight loss will help prevent muscle loss and will increase your metabolic rate, this helps keep the weight off. When you get close to your ideal weight, loosen up your diet and begin to build muscle by continually overloading your muscle with resistance, this will help you enjoy a little freedom and still maintain the weight you lost.

☐**Get your cadio in.** Cardiorespiratory exercise (cardio) strengthens your heart and lungs, giving you more ability to absorb oxygen into your bloodstream. Get your heart rate up and breathe deeply every day and provide plenty of oxygen. Our bodies use a higher percentage of body fat for energy needs when we are in an aerobic state (meaning, with oxygen). So make sure you breathe deeply.

☐ **Be mindful of your environment.** When exercising in hot weather or high altitudes, lower your intensity and increase your water consumption.

☐ **Use timeless nutrition information.**

☐ **Choosing to Give up a food item.** If you decide to give up a food item you enjoy because it's not helping you, expect to go through a grieving process.

☐ **Get your priorities straight.** Eat food because your body needs the nourishment. Your body is hungry for nutrients (water, protein, carbohydrate, fat, fiber, vitamins, and minerals). If you don't provide your body with the necessary nutrients, it will tell you via hunger that it needs certain nutrients. I recommend you start with the nutrient that makes up the majority of your body, water. It's wise to eliminate this zero calorie nutrient first. When you feel hunger, drink a glass of water and wait ten minutes. If you still feel hungry, enjoy a meal off of your kitchen's menu. Include the rest of the nutrients in each meal thereby giving your body what it needs.

☐ **O.W.N. your lifestyle.** Give your body Oxygen, Water, and Nutrients. Be responsible for what you do. If you eat the wrong foods, consume more calories than you burn, and don't exercise it will be difficult to lose fat.

☐**Stick to your plan** and eat logically, especially when you don't feel like it.

☐**A calorie is like an inch.** A calorie (like an inch) is the unit we use to measure the amount of energy in our food. Body fat is where we store excess energy for future use. So make sure you are at a calorie deficit meaning you burn more calories than you consume and not the other way around. Your body will always try to balance energy. If you only consume fewer calories to lose weight, you'll have to continually lower calories to lose weight. It's best to put your focus on using calories (exercising) while keeping calorie consumption under control. Exercising helps you manage carbohydrate metabolism and gives you an opportunity to build muscle, which makes weight loss more sustainable and less frustrating.

☐**The ideal meal.** A meal should consist of lean protein, complex carbohydrate, healthy fat, and fiber. A protein, carbohydrate, fat, and fiber in every meal.

☐**Eat regularly.** Ideally, you should eat every 3 to 4 hours, which equate to 4 to 5 meals a day. Never skip a meal and eat the same amount of calories in each meal. You can include 1 or 2 small 100 calorie meals to eat when you are busy. Eating in this manner helps keep your metabolism active.

☐**Enjoy your food.** Choose healthful foods you could enjoy for a lifetime. Take the foods you already enjoy and make them healthy meals. It's important to educate our taste buds or acquire the taste of healthy food in the same way many of us have done with alcohol. Be open-minded and try new foods with a curious mindset. It won't take long to enjoy these wonderful foods. A little secret. When food's in your mouth, and you're chewing, put the fork down and pay attention to the taste and the areas of your tongue being excited. This is how you educate your palate (taste buds).

☐ **Season your food.** Use salt, pepper, herbs, and spices. Create delicious dry rubs, marinades, and salsas to make your meals enjoyable.

☐ **Eat slowly.** Eating slow helps you taste and enjoy your food. Eating slow also helps with digestion and gives you an opportunity to listen to your body. Listen to what your gut is telling you.

☐ **Clean out your cupboards.** Donate food that's not helpful. Out of sight, is more likely, out of mind.

☐ **Be aware of what you put into your body.** Educate yourself about what's healthy. Read books, take classes on nutrition, cooking and exercising. Hire a dietitian, personal trainer, and talk to your doctor.

☐ **Search out and find healthy meals you like.** Buy a healthy cookbook, talk to friends, turn recipes that you already know into healthy meals. Start with a few days worth of meals and gradually add a few meals a week until you feel you have a good recipe base for your kitchen's menu. Create a plan or menu using the recipe base you've created. Create a shopping list using this week's plan, buy the ingredients and execute your plan.

☐ **Read nutrition and ingredient labels.** When you read a food label, you should be able to recognize and buy the ingredients. An ingredient label should look like a list of ingredients for a recipe. Your food and ingredient label should be simple.

☐ **Portion control.** You can eat your favorite foods, although it may be a smaller portion. Use small plates, and silverware, this helps with the visual. When you go out to eat, order a normal meal and eat only the amount that meets your calorie needs. Create leftovers and eat them later as a quick meal (put away leftovers before you finish your meal, don't let them sit in front of you). Drink a tall glass of water before a meal. It'll help you get this important nutrient and be fuller going into your meal. Eat a light salad as part of your meal, and get color into your diet, this will aid digestion for the meal and is a low-calorie way of helping you feel like you're eating enough food.

☐ **Take a multivitamin daily.** A multivitamin will help fill in any nutritional gaps that may be in your diet.

☐ **Never give up on YOU. Believe in yourself.**

Determining Calories in Food

Method 1

Read nutrition label on packages.

Always use this method.

It's very important to know what is in your food.

Method 2

Input food into a diet monitoring application.

This method is very accurate and can help
educate you on how much to eat. This method
takes daily work to input your food.

Method 3

Find or create meals that fit your, per meal, calorie goal.
The purpose of this method is to create a menu with
recipes for your kitchen. This method takes a few weeks
of work but will leave you educated with a variety of
meals that will help you in your journey to lose weight.

Method 4

Use an educated guess. (err on the side of caution)
This method, although less accurate and best used after
educating yourself for a few weeks, will be very useful
in the long run. Measure and weigh your food with
measuring cups, spoons and a scale. You can speed up
this process by measuring and weighing out all common
foods items you will eat. Spread them out on a table to
create a visual of what 100 calories looks like. Knowing
what 100 calories looks like will make guessing easier
and more accurate.

Process Oriented Fitness Related Goals.

- To get better at cooking health food
- To get better at running
- To get better at weightlifting
- To get better at yoga
- To get better at pilates
- To get better at swimming
- To get better at biking
- To get better at mountain biking
- To get better at martial arts
- To get better at dancing
- To get better at functional fitness
- To get better at skiing
- To get better at surfing
- To get better at skateboarding
- To get better at exercising
- To create your kitchens menu w/recipes and pics
- To create a healthy diet w/lots of variety
- To create my own periodized fitness program
- To create a cookbook
- To get off _blank_ medication
- To...

24 ways to burn 500 calories

- Jog for 60 min.
- Walk with a purpose for 120 min. (2 hours)
- Do Yoga for 120 min.
- Do Pilates for 100 min.
- Swim laps for 60 minutes.
- Bike riding with a purpose for 60 min.
- Mountain bike for 60 min.
- Circuit training for 60 min.
- High-intensity interval training for 50 min.
- Weightlifting (moderate) for 100 min.
- Practice martial arts for 50 min.
- Dance for 100 min.
- Ski, snowboard for 70 min.
- Do calisthenics (vigorously) for 60 min.
- Play a basketball game for 60 min.
- Play a football game for 60 min.
- Play volleyball for 60 min.
- Garden or do yard work for 160 min.
- Hike for 80 min.
- Play soccer for 70 min.
- Play tennis for 70 min.
- Do elliptical for 60 min.
- Do aerobics for 55 min.
- Do tai chi for 120 min.

Take the Journey

Do the 6 week challenge
and change your lifestyle.

The 6 Week Challenge

Welcome to the 6 week challenge and congradulations on your decision to change your life for the better. In this 6 week challenge you will make plans, create meals, and find exercises to help you lose weight. This will create the foundation for a healthy life-style. If you apply yourself and use this tool, you will produce results.

Follow the steps below and change your life-style.

Step 1: Take massive action and get the ball rolling
Start this journey by completing pages 73 through 79. Commit, set goals, know your numbers and take action.

Step 2: Make a plan and take daily action
Before the week starts plan your meals and when you will exercise. This step will get easier after completing step 3 for a few weeks. In the mean time do your best, keep to your calorie goal, and exercise daily.

Step 3: Do the weekly work to keep the ball rolling
Every week you will need to find two meals for each category (breakfast, lunch, dinner, and appetizer). Also you will need to find or create one workout routine each week. At the end of the 6 weeks you will have created a road map for life long success. This road map is the foundation for you to have a fit and healthy body.

The Commitment

It's time to make a commitment you won't let yourself back out of. Getting leverage on yourself, taking immediate action and showing perseverance will be your sign of a solid commitment. Remember, if you water your plan with daily action, you will produce fruit.

I am committing to losing _____ pounds.
By ___/ ___ / 20____. (Ideally 1-2 pounds per week)

Why must you lose weight? (Your Stick)

_____

How is the stick, that's hitting you, hurting you?

_____
_____

How will taking action, to get away from that stick, benefit you now?

_____
_____

Important: It's important to know what you want to achieve but this should not be your focus. Instead, focus on (visualize) the actions you have to take. When in the moment of picturing yourself taking action, it should feel good, achievable, something you can do. Focus on changing your behaviors, and you will change your life.

Goal Setting Workshop

Below, write your outcome goal from the previous page. Outcome goals give you direction, like saying, I want to see the statue of liberty. How you get there (be it walk, drive or fly) is what the process goal is all about.

Outcome goal

I will lose _____ pounds by ____ / ____ / 20____.

Your process goal is your carrot and a vehicle to help you achieve your outcome goal. It defines your daily actions and bridges the gap between the outcome you want and the lifestyle you are creating. It will create the "I am" or "I have" in your life. Choosing a process goal you truly want is important because it will be something you identify as. Example: If you get better at cooking, you become a good cook. It's time to choose a carrot. What do you want to have? Who do want to become? What do you want to get better at? pg. 69

Process Goal

I will get better at _____ and

every day I will _____

in order to get better at it.

Time to Take Action

Now that you are committed and have a process goal, it's time to take action. Do something right now towards your goal. Write this action below, put down this book and go do it. This should feel slightly uncomfortable.

_____

_____

_____

_____

Now you have got the ball rolling, build on this success, and strengthen your motivation to succeed. Write down two actions (one food, one fitness) you will do tomorrow and when you will do them. You should feel pressure, push through it.

Action 1 _____

Will be done by ____:____ am/pm ___/ ___/ 20___

Action 2 _____

Will be done by ____:____ am/pm ___/ ___/ 20___

Attitude Check

An optimistic, I will, attitude is an absolute must when we strive to change who we are to who we want to be. What kind of attitude do you hold? What beliefs are holding you back? (Check each box that apply)

- ☐ Are you willing to take action now?
- ☐ Will you confront the lies you tell yourself?
- ☐ Will you focus on your behaviors?
- ☐ Do you believe in yourself?
- ☐ Will you learn from your failures and grow?
- ☐ Are you willing to ask for help?
- ☐ Will you be patient with expectations?
- ☐ Are you enthusiastic about this journey?
- ☐ Will you welcome challenges?
- ☐ Are you willing to change?
- ☐ Do you need to change?
- ☐ Are you willing to make mistakes?
- ☐ Are you willing to exercise?
- ☐ Are you willing to eat healthily?
- ☐ Will you focus on what you can do?
- ☐ Will you focus on what you can have?
- ☐ Can you see yourself being successful?
- ☐ Can you ignore the naysayers?

Be honest.
If you have trouble checking a box, explore why.

The Starting Line

Resting Fitness Information
Name:_____ Date:_____
Age:___ Height:___ Weight:____ Ideal Weight:____
Resting HR:_____ BP:____/____ BMI:_____
Circumference Measurements
Chest:_____ Waist:_____ Hips:_____
Right Arm:_____ Left Arm:_____ Neck:_____
Right Thigh:____ Left Thigh:____ Right Wrist:____
Right Calf:_____ Left Calf:_____ Left Wrist:_____
Waist ÷ Hips = Hip to Waist Ratio:_____
Body Composition
Weight:_____ *Body Fat%:_____%
Lean Mass:_____ lb. Fat Mass:_____ lb.
Weight - body fat % = Lean Mass pounds (lean)
Weight - lean mass = Fat Mass pounds (fat)

*Body fat percentage is approximately determined using many methods: digital scale with bioimpedance, skinfold caliper, hydrostatic tank, bod pod, or a DEXA scan. Most new digital scales can measure body fat %. It's not important which method you use. However, it is important to use the same procedure (before and after), same time (in the morning after a 12 hour fast), similar hydration level (clear urine) and no caffeine for 24 hours.

Fueling the Body

Top Secret!!! The first step in addressing your food is knowing about how many calories you burn per day. In the equations below, put in your lean mass (page 77) or body weight and use the charts to determine what you perceive your metabolism and current activity to be and complete the equation to get your daily calories.

Less accurate

Body weight **X 10** = Resting Metabolic Rate **(RMR)**

More accurate   **OR**

Lean Mass **X 10 + 500** = Restng Metabolic Rate **(RMR)**

RMR **X** Metabolic Factor **X** Activity Factor = Daily Calories

You burn about_____ calories per day.

Metabolic Factor	Metabolism Description
0.90	Super slow, very hard to lose weight
0.95	Slow metabolism, hard to lose weight
1	Normal, able to lose and gain weight
1.25	Fast metabolism, hard to gain weight
1.5	Super fast, very hard to gain weight

Activity Factor	Activity Description
1.2	Sedentary, little to no physical activity
1.3	Light physical activity, most days
1.5	Moderate structured exercise, 1-3 days per week
1.8	Hard structured exercise, 4-6 days per week
2	Very hard structured exercise, daily

Fueling Goal

Now that you know how many calories you burn in a day, you can calculate how many calories you need in each meal. Below complete the equations to get your daily calorie needs and then calculate how many calories you need to eat per meal.

Calculate Daily Calorie Goal
Choose one

Weight loss
Daily Calories - 500 = Daily Calorie Goal

Maintain Weight
Daily Calories + 0 = Daily Calorie Goal

Weight gain
Daily Calories + 500 = Daily Calorie Goal

Daily Calorie Goal_____

Calculate Calories per Meal

Choose the number of meals you will eat per day_____

Daily calorie goal ÷ Meals per day = Calories per meal

Calories per meal_____

Know you know how many calories you need for each meal, it's time to find meals to meet your calorie need. Start by finding two meals for each category and once or more a week add two meal to each category. Keep your diet interesting and have a variety of meals.

Breakfast Menu
Include a receipt for each meal.

Meals	Calories
1_____	
_____	____
2_____	
_____	____
3_____	
_____	____
4_____	
_____	____
5_____	
_____	____
6_____	
_____	____
7_____	
_____	____
8_____	
_____	____
9_____	
_____	____
10_____	
_____	____
11_____	
_____	____
12_____	
_____	____

Lunch Menu
Include a receipt for each meal.

Meals   Calories

1_____

_____   _____

2_____

_____   _____

3_____

_____   _____

4_____

_____   _____

5_____

_____   _____

6_____

_____   _____

7_____

_____   _____

8_____

_____   _____

9_____

_____   _____

10_____

_____   _____

11_____

_____   _____

12_____

_____   _____

Dinner Menu
Include a receipt for each meal.

Meals   Calories

1 _____

_____   _____

2 _____

_____   _____

3 _____

_____   _____

4 _____

_____   _____

5 _____

_____   _____

6 _____

_____   _____

7 _____

_____   _____

8 _____

_____   _____

9 _____

_____   _____

10 _____

_____   _____

11 _____

_____   _____

12 _____

_____   _____

Small Meal (appetizer) Menu
Include a receipt for each meal.

Meals   Calories

1_____

_____   _____

2_____

_____   _____

3_____

_____   _____

4_____

_____   _____

5_____

_____   _____

6_____

_____   _____

7_____

_____   _____

8_____

_____   _____

9_____

_____   _____

10_____

_____   _____

11_____

_____   _____

12_____

_____   _____

Exercise Routine 1

Exercise Name:	Training Type:
Exercise Focus:	Training Intensity: %

Warm-up: Duration:

	Strength Exercises	Set 1	Set 2	Set 3	Set 4	Set 5
		Weight Reps	Weight Reps	Weight Reps	Weight Reps	Weight Reps
		Weight Reps	Weight Reps	Weight Reps	Weight Reps	Weight Reps
		Weight Reps	Weight Reps	Weight Reps	Weight Reps	Weight Reps
		Weight Reps	Weight Reps	Weight Reps	Weight Reps	Weight Reps
		Weight Reps	Weight Reps	Weight Reps	Weight Reps	Weight Reps
		Weight Reps	Weight Reps	Weight Reps	Weight Reps	Weight Reps
		Weight Reps	Weight Reps	Weight Reps	Weight Reps	Weight Reps
		Weight Reps	Weight Reps	Weight Reps	Weight Reps	Weight Reps
		Weight Reps	Weight Reps	Weight Reps	Weight Reps	Weight Reps
		Weight Reps	Weight Reps	Weight Reps	Weight Reps	Weight Reps
		Weight Reps	Weight Reps	Weight Reps	Weight Reps	Weight Reps
		Weight Reps	Weight Reps	Weight Reps	Weight Reps	Weight Reps
		Weight Reps	Weight Reps	Weight Reps	Weight Reps	Weight Reps

Cardiovascular / Flexibility Exercise	Min./Intensity %	
	min.	%
	min.	%
	min.	%

Cool Down: Duration:

Exercise Routine 2

Exercise Name:	Training Type:
Exercise Focus:	Training Intensity: %
Warm-up:	Duration:

	Strength Exercises	Set 1	Set 2	Set 3	Set 4	Set 5
		Weight Reps	Weight Reps	Weight Reps	Weight Reps	Weight Reps
		Weight Reps	Weight Reps	Weight Reps	Weight Reps	Weight Reps
		Weight Reps	Weight Reps	Weight Reps	Weight Reps	Weight Reps
		Weight Reps	Weight Reps	Weight Reps	Weight Reps	Weight Reps
		Weight Reps	Weight Reps	Weight Reps	Weight Reps	Weight Reps
		Weight Reps	Weight Reps	Weight Reps	Weight Reps	Weight Reps
		Weight Reps	Weight Reps	Weight Reps	Weight Reps	Weight Reps
		Weight Reps	Weight Reps	Weight Reps	Weight Reps	Weight Reps
		Weight Reps	Weight Reps	Weight Reps	Weight Reps	Weight Reps
		Weight Reps	Weight Reps	Weight Reps	Weight Reps	Weight Reps
		Weight Reps	Weight Reps	Weight Reps	Weight Reps	Weight Reps
		Weight Reps	Weight Reps	Weight Reps	Weight Reps	Weight Reps
		Weight Reps	Weight Reps	Weight Reps	Weight Reps	Weight Reps
	Cardiovascular / Flexibility Exercise	Min./Intensity %				
		min.	%			
		min.	%			
		min.	%			

Cool Down:	Duration:

Exercise Routine 3

Exercise Name:	Training Type:
Exercise Focus:	Training Intensity: %
Warm-up:	Duration:

Strength Exercises	Set 1	Set 2	Set 3	Set 4	Set 5
	Weight Reps	Weight Reps	Weight Reps	Weight Reps	Weight Reps
	Weight Reps	Weight Reps	Weight Reps	Weight Reps	Weight Reps
	Weight Reps	Weight Reps	Weight Reps	Weight Reps	Weight Reps
	Weight Reps	Weight Reps	Weight Reps	Weight Reps	Weight Reps
	Weight Reps	Weight Reps	Weight Reps	Weight Reps	Weight Reps
	Weight Reps	Weight Reps	Weight Reps	Weight Reps	Weight Reps
	Weight Reps	Weight Reps	Weight Reps	Weight Reps	Weight Reps
	Weight Reps	Weight Reps	Weight Reps	Weight Reps	Weight Reps
	Weight Reps	Weight Reps	Weight Reps	Weight Reps	Weight Reps
	Weight Reps	Weight Reps	Weight Reps	Weight Reps	Weight Reps
	Weight Reps	Weight Reps	Weight Reps	Weight Reps	Weight Reps
	Weight Reps	Weight Reps	Weight Reps	Weight Reps	Weight Reps
	Weight Reps	Weight Reps	Weight Reps	Weight Reps	Weight Reps

Cardiovascular / Flexibility Exercise	Min./Intensity %	
	min.	%
	min.	%
	min.	%

Cool Down:	Duration:

Exercise Routine 4

Exercise Name:	Training Type:
Exercise Focus:	Training Intensity: %

Warm-up:		Duration:

	Strength Exercises	Set 1	Set 2	Set 3	Set 4	Set 5
		Weight Reps	Weight Reps	Weight Reps	Weight Reps	Weight Reps
		Weight Reps	Weight Reps	Weight Reps	Weight Reps	Weight Reps
		Weight Reps	Weight Reps	Weight Reps	Weight Reps	Weight Reps
		Weight Reps	Weight Reps	Weight Reps	Weight Reps	Weight Reps
		Weight Reps	Weight Reps	Weight Reps	Weight Reps	Weight Reps
		Weight Reps	Weight Reps	Weight Reps	Weight Reps	Weight Reps
		Weight Reps	Weight Reps	Weight Reps	Weight Reps	Weight Reps
		Weight Reps	Weight Reps	Weight Reps	Weight Reps	Weight Reps
		Weight Reps	Weight Reps	Weight Reps	Weight Reps	Weight Reps
		Weight Reps	Weight Reps	Weight Reps	Weight Reps	Weight Reps
		Weight Reps	Weight Reps	Weight Reps	Weight Reps	Weight Reps
		Weight Reps	Weight Reps	Weight Reps	Weight Reps	Weight Reps
		Weight Reps	Weight Reps	Weight Reps	Weight Reps	Weight Reps

Cardiovascular / Flexibility Exercise	Min./Intensity %	
	min.	%
	min.	%
	min.	%

Cool Down:	Duration:

Exercise Routine 5

Exercise Name:	Training Type:
Exercise Focus:	Training Intensity: %

Warm-up: Duration:

	Strength Exercises	Set 1	Set 2	Set 3	Set 4	Set 5
		Weight Reps	Weight Reps	Weight Reps	Weight Reps	Weight Reps
		Weight Reps	Weight Reps	Weight Reps	Weight Reps	Weight Reps
		Weight Reps	Weight Reps	Weight Reps	Weight Reps	Weight Reps
		Weight Reps	Weight Reps	Weight Reps	Weight Reps	Weight Reps
		Weight Reps	Weight Reps	Weight Reps	Weight Reps	Weight Reps
		Weight Reps	Weight Reps	Weight Reps	Weight Reps	Weight Reps
		Weight Reps	Weight Reps	Weight Reps	Weight Reps	Weight Reps
		Weight Reps	Weight Reps	Weight Reps	Weight Reps	Weight Reps
		Weight Reps	Weight Reps	Weight Reps	Weight Reps	Weight Reps
		Weight Reps	Weight Reps	Weight Reps	Weight Reps	Weight Reps
		Weight Reps	Weight Reps	Weight Reps	Weight Reps	Weight Reps
		Weight Reps	Weight Reps	Weight Reps	Weight Reps	Weight Reps
		Weight Reps	Weight Reps	Weight Reps	Weight Reps	Weight Reps
	Cardiovascular / Flexibility Exercise	Min./Intensity %				
		min. %				
		min. %				
		min. %				

Cool Down:	Duration:

Exercise Routine 6

Exercise Name:	Training Type:
Exercise Focus:	Training Intensity: %

Warm-up: Duration:

	Strength Exercises	Set 1	Set 2	Set 3	Set 4	Set 5
		Weight Reps	Weight Reps	Weight Reps	Weight Reps	Weight Reps
		Weight Reps	Weight Reps	Weight Reps	Weight Reps	Weight Reps
		Weight Reps	Weight Reps	Weight Reps	Weight Reps	Weight Reps
		Weight Reps	Weight Reps	Weight Reps	Weight Reps	Weight Reps
		Weight Reps	Weight Reps	Weight Reps	Weight Reps	Weight Reps
		Weight Reps	Weight Reps	Weight Reps	Weight Reps	Weight Reps
		Weight Reps	Weight Reps	Weight Reps	Weight Reps	Weight Reps
		Weight Reps	Weight Reps	Weight Reps	Weight Reps	Weight Reps
		Weight Reps	Weight Reps	Weight Reps	Weight Reps	Weight Reps
		Weight Reps	Weight Reps	Weight Reps	Weight Reps	Weight Reps
		Weight Reps	Weight Reps	Weight Reps	Weight Reps	Weight Reps
		Weight Reps	Weight Reps	Weight Reps	Weight Reps	Weight Reps
		Weight Reps	Weight Reps	Weight Reps	Weight Reps	Weight Reps

Cardiovascular / Flexibility Exercise	Min./Intensity %	
	min.	%
	min.	%
	min.	%

Cool Down:	Duration:

Week 1 plan

Build your behavior changing muscle.
Decide what you will do, then go do it.

I will get better at _____and
everyday I will_____.

Monday   Exercise & Food
Exercise_____When_____Duration_____
Meal 1_____ _____
Meal 2_____ _____
Meal 3_____ _____
Meal 4_____ _____
Meal 5_____ _____

Tuesday   Exercise & Food
Exercise_____When_____Duration_____
Meal 1_____ _____
Meal 2_____ _____
Meal 3_____ _____
Meal 4_____ _____
Meal 5_____ _____

Wednesday   Exercise & Food
Exercise_____When_____Duration_____
Meal 1_____ _____
Meal 2_____ _____
Meal 3_____ _____
Meal 4_____ _____
Meal 5_____ _____

Thursday <u>Exercise & Food</u>
Exercise_____ When_____ Duration_____
Meal 1_____ _____
Meal 2_____ _____
Meal 3_____ _____
Meal 4_____ _____
Meal 5_____ _____

Friday <u>Exercise & Food</u>
Exercise_____ When_____ Duration_____
Meal 1_____ _____
Meal 2_____ _____
Meal 3_____ _____
Meal 4_____ _____
Meal 5_____ _____

Saturday <u>Exercise & Food</u>
Exercise_____ When_____ Duration_____
Meal 1_____ _____
Meal 2_____ _____
Meal 3_____ _____
Meal 4_____ _____
Meal 5_____ _____

Sunday <u>Exercise & Food</u>
Exercise_____ When_____ Duration_____
Meal 1_____ _____
Meal 2_____ _____
Meal 3_____ _____
Meal 4_____ _____
Meal 5_____ _____

Week 2 plan
Build your behavior changing muscle.
Decide what you will do, then go do it.

I will get better at _____and
everyday I will_____.

Monday   Exercise & Food
Exercise_____ When_____ Duration_____
Meal 1_____ _____
Meal 2_____ _____
Meal 3_____ _____
Meal 4_____ _____
Meal 5_____ _____

Tuesday   Exercise & Food
Exercise_____ When_____ Duration_____
Meal 1_____ _____
Meal 2_____ _____
Meal 3_____ _____
Meal 4_____ _____
Meal 5_____ _____

Wednesday   Exercise & Food
Exercise_____ When_____ Duration_____
Meal 1_____ _____
Meal 2_____ _____
Meal 3_____ _____
Meal 4_____ _____
Meal 5_____ _____

Thursday Exercise & Food
Exercise_____ When_____ Duration_____
Meal 1_____ _____
Meal 2_____ _____
Meal 3_____ _____
Meal 4_____ _____
Meal 5_____ _____

Friday Exercise & Food
Exercise_____ When_____ Duration_____
Meal 1_____ _____
Meal 2_____ _____
Meal 3_____ _____
Meal 4_____ _____
Meal 5_____ _____

Saturday Exercise & Food
Exercise_____ When_____ Duration_____
Meal 1_____ _____
Meal 2_____ _____
Meal 3_____ _____
Meal 4_____ _____
Meal 5_____ _____

Sunday Exercise & Food
Exercise_____ When_____ Duration_____
Meal 1_____ _____
Meal 2_____ _____
Meal 3_____ _____
Meal 4_____ _____
Meal 5_____ _____

Week 3 plan

Build your behavior changing muscle.
Decide what you will do, then go do it.

I will get better at _____and
everyday I will_____.

Monday   <u>Exercise & Food</u>
Exercise_____When_____Duration_____
Meal 1_____ _____
Meal 2_____ _____
Meal 3_____ _____
Meal 4_____ _____
Meal 5_____ _____

Tuesday   <u>Exercise & Food</u>
Exercise_____When_____Duration_____
Meal 1_____ _____
Meal 2_____ _____
Meal 3_____ _____
Meal 4_____ _____
Meal 5_____ _____

Wednesday   <u>Exercise & Food</u>
Exercise_____When_____Duration_____
Meal 1_____ _____
Meal 2_____ _____
Meal 3_____ _____
Meal 4_____ _____
Meal 5_____ _____

Thursday　　　<u>Exercise & Food</u>
Exercise_____ When_____Duration_____
Meal 1_____ _____
Meal 2_____ _____
Meal 3_____ _____
Meal 4_____ _____
Meal 5_____ _____

Friday　　　<u>Exercise & Food</u>
Exercise_____ When_____Duration_____
Meal 1_____ _____
Meal 2_____ _____
Meal 3_____ _____
Meal 4_____ _____
Meal 5_____ _____

Saturday　　　<u>Exercise & Food</u>
Exercise_____ When_____Duration_____
Meal 1_____ _____
Meal 2_____ _____
Meal 3_____ _____
Meal 4_____ _____
Meal 5_____ _____

Sunday　　　<u>Exercise & Food</u>
Exercise_____ When_____Duration_____
Meal 1_____ _____
Meal 2_____ _____
Meal 3_____ _____
Meal 4_____ _____
Meal 5_____ _____

Week 4 plan
Build your behavior changing muscle.
Decide what you will do, then go do it.

I will get better at _____and
everyday I will_____.

Monday   Exercise & Food
Exercise_____When_____Duration_____
Meal 1_____ _____
Meal 2_____ _____
Meal 3_____ _____
Meal 4_____ _____
Meal 5_____ _____

Tuesday   Exercise & Food
Exercise_____When_____Duration_____
Meal 1_____ _____
Meal 2_____ _____
Meal 3_____ _____
Meal 4_____ _____
Meal 5_____ _____

Wednesday   Exercise & Food
Exercise_____When_____Duration_____
Meal 1_____ _____
Meal 2_____ _____
Meal 3_____ _____
Meal 4_____ _____
Meal 5_____ _____

Thursday   <u>Exercise & Food</u>
Exercise_____ When_____Duration_____
Meal 1_____ _____
Meal 2_____ _____
Meal 3_____ _____
Meal 4_____ _____
Meal 5_____ _____

Friday   <u>Exercise & Food</u>
Exercise_____ When_____Duration_____
Meal 1_____ _____
Meal 2_____ _____
Meal 3_____ _____
Meal 4_____ _____
Meal 5_____ _____

Saturday   <u>Exercise & Food</u>
Exercise_____ When_____Duration_____
Meal 1_____ _____
Meal 2_____ _____
Meal 3_____ _____
Meal 4_____ _____
Meal 5_____ _____

Sunday   <u>Exercise & Food</u>
Exercise_____ When_____Duration_____
Meal 1_____ _____
Meal 2_____ _____
Meal 3_____ _____
Meal 4_____ _____
Meal 5_____ _____

Week 5 plan
Build your behavior changing muscle.
Decide what you will do, then go do it.

I will get better at _____and
everyday I will_____.

Monday   Exercise & Food
Exercise_____ When_____ Duration_____
Meal 1_____ _____
Meal 2_____ _____
Meal 3_____ _____
Meal 4_____ _____
Meal 5_____ _____

Tuesday   Exercise & Food
Exercise_____ When_____ Duration_____
Meal 1_____ _____
Meal 2_____ _____
Meal 3_____ _____
Meal 4_____ _____
Meal 5_____ _____

Wednesday   Exercise & Food
Exercise_____ When_____ Duration_____
Meal 1_____ _____
Meal 2_____ _____
Meal 3_____ _____
Meal 4_____ _____
Meal 5_____ _____

Thursday   <u>Exercise & Food</u>

Exercise_____When_____Duration_____

Meal 1_____ _____

Meal 2_____ _____

Meal 3_____ _____

Meal 4_____ _____

Meal 5_____ _____

Friday   <u>Exercise & Food</u>

Exercise_____When_____Duration_____

Meal 1_____ _____

Meal 2_____ _____

Meal 3_____ _____

Meal 4_____ _____

Meal 5_____ _____

Saturday   <u>Exercise & Food</u>

Exercise_____When_____Duration_____

Meal 1_____ _____

Meal 2_____ _____

Meal 3_____ _____

Meal 4_____ _____

Meal 5_____ _____

Sunday   <u>Exercise & Food</u>

Exercise_____When_____Duration_____

Meal 1_____ _____

Meal 2_____ _____

Meal 3_____ _____

Meal 4_____ _____

Meal 5_____ _____

Week 6 plan

Build your behavior changing muscle.
Decide what you will do, then go do it.

I will get better at _____and
everyday I will_____.

Monday   <u>Exercise & Food</u>
Exercise_____When_____Duration_____
Meal 1_____ _____
Meal 2_____ _____
Meal 3_____ _____
Meal 4_____ _____
Meal 5_____ _____

Tuesday   <u>Exercise & Food</u>
Exercise_____When_____Duration_____
Meal 1_____ _____
Meal 2_____ _____
Meal 3_____ _____
Meal 4_____ _____
Meal 5_____ _____

Wednesday   <u>Exercise & Food</u>
Exercise_____When_____Duration_____
Meal 1_____ _____
Meal 2_____ _____
Meal 3_____ _____
Meal 4_____ _____
Meal 5_____ _____

Thursday   Exercise & Food
Exercise_____When_____Duration_____
Meal 1_____ _____
Meal 2_____ _____
Meal 3_____ _____
Meal 4_____ _____
Meal 5_____ _____

Friday   Exercise & Food
Exercise_____When_____Duration_____
Meal 1_____ _____
Meal 2_____ _____
Meal 3_____ _____
Meal 4_____ _____
Meal 5_____ _____

Saturday   Exercise & Food
Exercise_____When_____Duration_____
Meal 1_____ _____
Meal 2_____ _____
Meal 3_____ _____
Meal 4_____ _____
Meal 5_____ _____

Sunday   Exercise & Food
Exercise_____When_____Duration_____
Meal 1_____ _____
Meal 2_____ _____
Meal 3_____ _____
Meal 4_____ _____
Meal 5_____ _____

Notes